PRAISE FOR

F THE FEVER

"Brisk, vivid, and all too relatable, Lon Wagner's *The Fever* transports modern pandemic survivors into the bedchambers, clinics, and graveyards of a thriving American port laid low by pestilence—and reflects on just how much and how little we've learned in the 170 years since."

—Earl Swift, author of *Hell Put to Shame: The 1921 Murder Farm Massacre and the Horror of America's Second Slavery*

"As suspenseful as it is moving, Lon Wagner's *The Fever* gives veterans of our modern-day pandemic a historic and page-turning primer on another outbreak that took place a century and a half ago. Fans of Geraldine Brooks's *Year of Wonders* and Hampton Sides's *In the Kingdom of Ice* will find much to admire in the voices of ordinary people who took on so many challenges in the face of grave danger and almost certain death. A riveting, meticulously researched account."

—Beth Macy, author of *Dopesick*

"In *The Fever*, Lon Wagner tells the awful story of an 1855 yellow fever epidemic in Tidewater, Virginia, one of the most catastrophic events in American history. This book is an important reminder of the ability of epidemic and pandemic threats to destabilize a society and threaten its security. We must also be mindful of how, because of modern-day climate change and urbanization, yellow fever remains a threat to the Southern US and could one day return."

—Peter Hotez, MD, PhD, dean, National School of Tropical Medicine at Baylor College of Medicine, endowed chair of Tropical Pediatrics, Texas Children's Hospital

"Richly reported and eloquently written, this true story transports readers back to 1855, into a raging epidemic that feels eerily prescient. Lon Wagner's *The Fever* is a tragic, triumphant tale of desperate people struggling to make sense of a deadly epidemic—and save themselves. Wagner reminds us that though progress has paved roads and pioneered vaccines, some people still use fear to justify prejudice, while others sacrifice themselves to save strangers."

—Lane DeGregory, winner of the Pulitzer Prize in feature writing

"Lon Wagner's compelling narrative brings to life the extraordinary courage and compassion faced by the residents of Norfolk and Portsmouth, Virginia, when confronted with a disease that may have been up to 100 times deadlier than COVID-19. *The Fever* is a story of resilience, generosity, and selflessness, as well as human frailty and fear, in the face of an unknown and relentless enemy. It is a gripping account honoring the indomitable human spirit and reminding us that the past is prologue."

—Ron Fricker, PhD, professor of statistics, author of
Monitoring the Health of Populations by Tracking Disease
Outbreaks: Saving Humanity from the Next Plague

"As a medical reporter at *USA Today*, I covered outbreaks of numerous mosquito-borne viruses—including West Nile, Zika, dengue, and chikungunya—but never with the rich narrative detail that Lon Wagner provides in this captivating history, which reads as much like a detective story as a work of nonfiction."

—Liz Szabo, independent health and science reporter

The Fever: The Most Fatal Plague in American History
by Lon Wagner

© Copyright 2024 Lon Wagner

979-8-88824-421-0

Published by

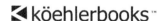 köehlerbooks™

3705 Shore Drive
Virginia Beach, VA 23455
800-435-4811
www.koehlerbooks.com

THE
FEVER

The Most Fatal Plague in American History

LON WAGNER

VIRGINIA BEACH
CAPE CHARLES

For my daughters, Ava, Sadie, and Lilla.
And for Bonnie.

TABLE OF CONTENTS

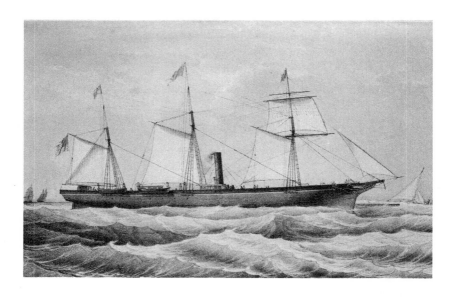

The steamship *Benjamin Franklin*. Credit: The Mariners' Museum and Park, Newport News, Virginia.

INTRODUCTION

I

N the summer of 1855, a virus stowed away on a ship and swept into two unsuspecting cities on the southern coast of Virginia. What happened over the next four months has no parallel in American history.

This virus let loose an epidemic more deadly than the Great Plague of London. It sent thousands of terrified people fleeing on steamships and rail cars, in horse-drawn carts, and on foot, carrying whatever they could. It wiped out entire families and forced burials in pits, with bodies stacked on top of each other like firewood. It orphaned children too young to know their own names.

Yellow fever spread from mosquitoes to people and back again, in an exponential loop. The more infected people, the more infected mosquitoes, and so on. This virus no longer afflicts the United States, though it continues to kill more than thirty thousand people in tropical climates each year. So, this story could have been viewed much like a period film—with rapt fascination, from the safety of a modern world.

Then came the winter of 2020, when a virus stowed away on airplanes and swept across the globe. What happened in the years after is different in some ways than what occurred in the summer of 1855—how the virus spread, the fatality rate, and how quickly science raced to find a way to tamp it down.

Yet the two are more similar than different, and that's because while technology advances, human nature remains the same. In 1855, as in 2020, people did not know much about how the virus spread or what was killing them. Panic and fear drove their behavior.

Those with means fled from the danger while those without faced the greatest risks. Many mocked the doctors who first called attention to the threat and scorned them for ruining the economy.

Though what you are about to read may seem farfetched, or exaggerated, every word is true. It happened. Then, it happened again.

CHAPTER ONE
A Big Mistake

I T was like this every summer. A ship would steam north from a Caribbean port, loaded with passengers, sugar, coffee, and fruit. At an American port, its crew would unload the cargo, its passengers would disperse into the town, and the rain barrels used for drinking water would be dumped out. All the fixings of a nineteenth-century outbreak stirred together in a city dense with people. In late May 1855, it looked a lot like that summer the ship would be the *Benjamin Franklin*, about to haul out of Saint Thomas. And it seemed like the port would be New York.

The *Benjamin Franklin* had been at anchor in the West Indies for much of that spring when crew members of nearly every ship in the harbor came down with yellow fever, a tropical disease that had plagued ships and port cities since Europeans began capturing people in Africa more than two hundred years earlier. *The Keystone* had lost six of its crew while in Saint Thomas, and another two died en route to New York.[1] Only after the devastation of the summer of 1855 would it become known that the *Franklin* had eight or nine cases aboard while docked in Saint Thomas that spring. On May 25, two days before the Franklin sailed north, Jonathan Bowen joined the crew as chief engineer.[2] Trouble immediately came his way. One of his firemen—the young men charged with shoveling coal into the engine's boilers—sought out the engineer. "He complained of pain in the head and also a pain in the small of his back," Bowen remembered. "His tongue was coated with a dark brown crust."[3]

Bowen sent for the captain. Captain John Byram came to see the fireman himself. It was critical to keep the information loop tight. No port would permit the *Franklin* to land with cases of yellow fever on board.

Byram handed Bowen a small bottle of grainy, white powder. Bowen removed the cork and gave the fireman a dose of calomel. That was the only thing Byram knew to use to cure a person of yellow fever. It was mercury chloride, both a poisonous chemical and a purgative, so it might cause a sick person to expel the toxins and recover. That was the theory anyway. More often than not, the drug made its victims purge so much that it drained them of fluids, setting them on the path to a miserable, toxic death. This time, the fireman survived, both the medicine and the virus.

Samuel Travers had also boarded the *Franklin* for the journey north. Travers lived and breathed salt water: He was a respected shipmaster from Taylor's Island, Maryland, a marshy part of the Eastern Shore that arched out into the Chesapeake Bay. He spent nearly every winter as a resident of Saint Thomas. Travers did not know about the fireman; in fact, he thought the *Franklin* was free of disease. He just wanted to get the heck away from Saint Thomas as soon as possible. After a horrendous epidemic that summer, Travers wrote to the committee that investigated its origin:

> "THE ISLAND at that time was distressingly sick with yellow fever. From a number of years' residence in the West Indies, I should certainly pronounce it yellow fever of the worst type."[4]

For two hundred years, Saint Thomas had been distressingly sick, or at least some level of sick, with the terrorizing disease. It was no exaggeration to say that the island's sickness foretold a great deal of risk for the entire Western Hemisphere. The West Indies, specifically the tiny Saint Thomas harbor, was the hub through which nearly all shipped goods and many people had to pass. Steamers ran direct routes from Saint Thomas to Baltimore, Philadelphia, New York, and Boston, along with the thriving midsized ports along the East Coast, including Savannah, Georgia; Charleston, South Carolina; and Norfolk, Virginia. In the mid-1800s, with only a piecemeal rail network, shipping access equaled prestige and the East Coast port cities were Main Street, USA. Every day, ships sailed into Saint Thomas with loads of captive people from West Africa. After being beaten and dragged from their homes in Africa and penned up in filthy conditions in the holds of ships, the captives were either sold into slavery in the West Indies—where their masters worked them to the brink of death on sugar, cotton, and fruit farms—or kept on the ship to be sold up north.

Yellow fever was a curse of this international slave trade. Before Europeans began capturing people in Africa and shipping them like cargo across the ocean, the virus had long circulated in dense jungles. It traveled as mosquitoes flew, and mosquitoes don't fly very far. As soon as ships began hauling people from West Africa to the Caribbean and European colonies in the 1600s, yellow fever became a constant threat to any port where ships docked. It would stalk East Coast and Mississippi River cities for the next three hundred years.

Saint Thomas had attained its internationally outsized status when the Danes, its colonial rulers, granted a monopoly to the Dutch West India Company to set up a trading station there. The island became the nerve center for anything being transported from Africa, the Brazilian coast, all the East Coast ports, and those along the Mississippi, New Orleans, and Memphis. As a *New York Times* correspondent marveled: "The whole world seems to have tacitly agreed that Saint Thomas should be the depot of West Indian commerce. They have made it the

rendezvous of the largest fleet of commercial steamers in the world."
It was puzzling, he wrote, because other islands had harbors in equally
good locations, with much better reputations for good health.

Saint Thomas was a cramped town, with mountains that pinched
homes, shops, and bars hard against the harbor. So many pubs
crammed the streets around the port that sea hands in the 1600s
dubbed the burg "Taphus," or Tap House. The densely packed town
of eleven thousand and the constant arrival of new people jammed
into dark ship quarters made it the perfect place for circulating viruses,
whether typhoid, cholera, or malaria. But the most feared disease was
yellow fever, an illness so terrifying that it sent people fleeing from
their homes and chased entire populations from cities. Saint Thomas
was a major incubator of this annual, never-ending cycle of sickness.
Every spring and summer, an armada of ticking biological bombs
departed its harbor and headed for northern ports.

"The news from this little island is generally confined to deaths
from yellow fever—sometimes more, sometimes less—but always
sufficiently numerous to terrify the unacclimated," the *Times*
correspondent wrote. "No northern vessel can enter port and discharge
her cargo without losing one or more of her crew."

People were hunted by an invisible virus. They didn't know what
to run from. Doctors didn't know how to treat it. Scientific discovery
moved, at its fastest, on a timeline marked in decades; at its slowest,
on a pace of centuries. With no knowledge, no help, and no hope,
people stood by and watched the fever torture family and friends to
the depths of misery.

A victim's torment starts three to six days after being bitten by an
infected mosquito. Yellow fever comes on like a lot of illnesses, with
a headache, a pesky backache, muscle pain, a fever, and vomiting.
And that's a mild case. For some, the body fights off the virus and
symptoms fade after three or four days. For others, the battle has just
begun. They get a whiff of hope that it's over, that they've survived.
Then the fever enters a toxic phase. The virus attacks the kidneys.

It breaches the liver and shuts it down. The person's skin turns an ashen yellow.[5]

If a person dies right then, it would be merciful. But this virus shows no mercy. After more than a week of torment, the victim throws up and keeps throwing up. What comes out looks like digested coffee grounds speckled with red dots. Called black vomit, it's not vomit at all but the byproduct of internal hemorrhaging. Few people live after black vomit. In the 1700s and 1800s, it was nature's version of bioterror: When residents saw others with black vomit, they abandoned dying loved ones; and neighboring cities banned people traveling from infected areas fearing they'd bring the disease with them.

Even before yellow fever had a name, it was throttling the British colonies. In 1668, vicious fevers erupted in Philadelphia and New York, and those cities would suffer similar attacks repeatedly over the next century and a half: Philadelphia, twenty times; New York, fifteen; Boston, eight; Baltimore, seven. Charleston endured more than two dozen outbreaks. Norfolk, and always by extension its sister city, Portsmouth[6], had been hit as early as 1737 and again in 1741 and 1743, and notably almost every year of the first decade of the 1800s, and again in 1826.[7]

It took more than a century for people to have a hunch that the virus was coming from Africa. With the colonies in demand of more slave labor for expanding plantations, the European traders delved deeper inland in West Africa. In 1768, French traders forayed three hundred miles up the Senegal River seeking better prices for captive Africans than they could get closer to port. When they got back to the coast and boarded, the fever swept across the ship.[8]

Sir Walter Scott and many other writers played up the fears of ships infected with yellow fever, or "yellow jack." In the legend of the *Flying Dutchman*, harbor after harbor refuses to allow the ship to dock for fear of what is on board. Eventually, the crew dies. The unmanned vessel is doomed to roam forever as a ghost ship around the

Cape of Good Hope. The horror was rooted in truth. Surely, things could breed in droplets of rainwater in crevices on old wooden ships. Certainly, the crew, passengers, captives, and the entire ship could become a giant petri dish for transmitting and breeding disease on the way across the ocean.

In any given summer, no one knew which ship would have sick crew carrying the virus, which port city it would dock in, or how many residents in that city at that moment were immune. Every port city was on the lookout, every year, for something that might trigger an epidemic.

The *Benjamin Franklin* sailed out of Saint Thomas on May 27, 1855, carrying crates of oranges, grapefruits, and pineapples. More than fifty pleasure passengers also traveled on the *Franklin*, a stunning ship commissioned four years earlier for the glamorous job of running tourists on the weekly trip from Philadelphia to Boston. It exuded elegance, with glistening wooden sides and deck, three masts—fore, middle, and aft—along with a massive exhaust pipe at midship to vent smoke from the coal-fired boilers below. When the *Franklin* was under full sail, with its rigging cutting in sharp angles from the masts to the deck, she was regal. In slack air, her two three-hundred-fifty-horsepower steam engines carried the load.[9] Despite her handsome looks and power, a perplexing amount of trouble nearly always turned up in her wake.

The Philadelphia-to-Boston route soon went bankrupt. The *Franklin's* owners sent the ship to the Caribbean and South America to hustle up work. By September 1854, it was docked in a New York shipyard, reportedly being fitted with ten thirty-two-pound cannons. That gun packed about ten pounds of gunpowder to fire a thirty-two-pound ball and enough ammo to engage a small navy. It was rumored that the *Franklin* and an armed-to-the-teeth ship named the *Catharine Augusta* would soon be the phalanx of an invasion of Venezuela. General José Antonio Páez had led Venezuela to independence in 1830 but had been forced out of power in the 1840s and exiled to New York. Word had it that Páez aimed to overthrow the Venezuelan dictator, who had ousted him, and retake the country. But when authorities searched the *Franklin* in New York, they did not find anything awry. The ship was cleared to sail and set out for Saint Thomas on September 19. The *Franklin* arrived at the harbor ten days later, suspiciously, with the heavily armed *Catharine Augusta*.[10]

They were at first ordered to leave the port. No one there wanted trouble. The *New York Times* reported that the arrival of the two ships "created considerable speculation as to their intentions." It was curious. Both ships had more men on board than any cargo ship would ever need. But because the *Augusta* had been damaged en route, authorities allowed it to dock for repairs, and the *Franklin* was permitted to tag along. Rumors aside, the *Franklin* never helped invade Venezuela.

By January 1855, the Royal Mail Steam Company chartered the *Franklin* to engage in what should have been the mundane work of ferrying English mail and passengers from Saint Thomas to other islands. The *Times* reported on an incident as the ship was making its rounds: "The American steamer *Benjamin Franklin* was fired into by the authorities of the island when leaving port, one ball passing through a state-room in which were an English lady and child." Authorities figured the *Franklin* was up to something and cited it for not having a pass to travel at night.[11] The *Franklin* lost its mail-courier job, and the ship idled for months in sickly Saint Thomas during the winter of 1855.

Two days after it pulled out of the West Indies in late May, a boy who worked in the mess hall reported a fever, chills, headache, and body aches. Bowen, the engineer, gave him a dose of calomel, but it didn't work. Three days later, the boy died. Bowen and the crew were careful to not let the passengers find out. That night, they wrapped the boy in a bedsheet, carried his body to the ship's railing, and dropped him into the ocean. They never reported his death.

The *Franklin* continued north, skirting past Savannah and Charleston, where another ship had unleashed an epidemic the year before. That fever slayed more than one thousand in Savannah and another six hundred twenty-seven in Charleston. Two years earlier, in 1853, a devastating epidemic had killed eight thousand in New Orleans. In Virginia, residents feared that, year by year, yellow fever was working its way up the coast.

But Captain Byram and the *Franklin* faced a more immediate problem. The ship had begun taking on water. Byram told the engineer to spur his firemen to heave coal into the boiler faster to keep the steamship stoked on a dead sprint for New York. At the same time, panicked and desperate for crew, he enlisted the male pleasure passengers to work the bilge pumps in the hold. It was chaos. They stood in seawater, teeming with disgusting detritus. The faster the ship went, the more seawater poured through the cracks around the masts. The more water, the faster the tourists tried to pump. Then a fireman died, showing all the signs of yellow fever.

For three days and nights, passengers and crew worked the pumps to keep the ship from sinking, but the *Franklin* could not outrace its fate.[12] By the time the ship skirted Cape Hatteras, Byram had given up on the run to New York. He guided the *Franklin* west toward land, aiming for Cape Henry, Virginia, and through the confluence of the Atlantic Ocean, the Chesapeake Bay, and the James River.

Every mariner for the past two hundred years was familiar with where those three bodies of water swirled together, called Hampton Roads. Byram also knew that his last hope lay around one more bend in the river, the ship repair yards of Norfolk and Portsmouth. Those cities were wedged in the far southeast corner of Virginia—Norfolk squeezed onto one bank of the Elizabeth River, Portsmouth to the south on the other side. Even today, a person can stand at water's edge of either city and clearly see the other. The *Franklin* had waylaid there two years earlier. Steaming out of New Orleans bound for New York, she'd run out of coal and sailed into Norfolk to refill.[13]

This time, before they entered the harbor, the passengers petitioned Byram with a demand. They'd had enough. They'd seen enough. They wanted off the ship. So there, in the choppy open waters where the currents mixed and the tides pulled, the crew helped the well-off but desperate tourists climb over the edge of the *Franklin*. Another vessel powered close as the crew hastily lashed the two ships together. It was a harrowing, death-defying moment. With the ships rocking, the passengers hopped aboard and the second ship steamed away.

Byram guided the *Franklin*, still taking on water, toward Norfolk and Portsmouth. Just upriver from the population centers of the two towns, he dropped anchor at the "quarantine grounds," where the *Franklin* would remain until the city's health officer could inspect it for disease.

Many cities now had quarantine grounds. No one knew how people got yellow fever, where it came from, or what transmitted it, but they'd seen enough to know it often broke out soon after certain ships came into harbor. As a precaution, port cities required ships to anchor off to one side of the shipping channel, usually about a mile upriver from the city's center. The Norfolk health officer, a doctor appointed by the City Council, had to inspect a ship and pronounce it free of disease before it was allowed to dock. The sister cities had established quarantine grounds, just offshore of Fort Norfolk, an outpost set up as part of George Washington's maritime frontier. With its US flag out on the point, the fort was long considered the mark at which a ship had entered the Norfolk harbor.

On that evening of June 6, 1855, the *Franklin*'s exhausted crew sprang into action. Under a half-moon's light, they readied the ship for inspection. They scrubbed the deck, emptied the cargo hold, and chucked rotting fruit over the side into the Elizabeth River. Pressed for time, they wrapped the body of the dead fireman in bedsheets and heaved him into the river, too. The next day, the first summerlike day of the year, the thermometer hit eighty-six degrees.[14] A thick breeze oozed from the west as the health inspector ferried to the quarantine grounds. As Doctor Robert Gordon came nearer, the ship's gleaming wooden sides mirrored the clouds in the sky.

Quarantine grounds were often the setting for a cat-and-mouse showdown. A health officer had to walk a tightrope between allowing commerce to continue and preventing a ship from importing the seeds of a deadly epidemic. And a ship's captain, by trade, was a professional liar.

The captain's job was to keep the ship moving toward its destination, while a port's health officer was as much an obstacle to progress as a leaking ship or a storm at sea. In Norfolk, Gordon had boarded scores of ships over the years. If he suspected contagion aboard, he'd order the ship to remain anchored in the wide part of the channel and to fly a yellow quarantine flag from its mast until it could be reinspected and found not to be a threat. With their journeys halted, passengers would disembark and demand refunds. Fruit would ripen, then rot, and have to be dumped overboard.

Decades earlier, in 1793, ships of refugees from Santo Domingo, the capital of the Dominican Republic, began arriving in Philadelphia. Those enslaved on the island had rioted against their French masters, and a series of bloody massacres followed. Refugees poured into Philadelphia, some bringing their enslaved with them, more than two thousand people in all. Residents welcomed them and raised more than sixteen thousand dollars to help house and feed the immigrants. But a few weeks later, a virus began to overtake Philadelphia, at the time the country's largest city and its capital. As people began dying, President George Washington and the Congress fled for safety, and more than four thousand of those who stayed behind died. Doctor Benjamin Rush, a signer of the Declaration of Independence, correctly identified yellow fever as the culprit. He surmised that it had originated from rotting coffee on a wharf—incorrectly, it turned out.[15]

During another yellow fever outbreak in 1853, the *Augusta* entered the New Orleans harbor after sailing up the Mississippi River with a second ship that had departed from Kingston, Jamaica, where yellow fever raged. Irish immigrants on the *Augusta* contracted yellow fever and ignited an epidemic that would kill forty-eight hundred people in New Orleans and another three thousand in nearby river towns.[16]

In late June the following year, 1854, a Danish ship called the *Charlotte Hague* arrived at Cockspur Inlet off Savannah, Georgia. The vessel had sailed from Cuba, where parts of the island were now infected with yellow fever. After visiting the ship several times to treat a sick captain and crew, Savannah's health officer thought it would be more convenient to transfer the men to a private hospital. Yellow fever spread throughout the city that August and September, killing more than six hundred. The ship never sailed all the way into the Savannah harbor.

Disease carried in by a ship could set a city back for years. When the afflicted place was in the South, Northern newspapers gleefully covered the tragedy with great sympathy and detail—barrels of ink and tons of newsprint devoted to not-so-subtly letting business owners understand the gamble they'd be taking if they wanted to expand to the South. There were plenty of diseases to fear: cholera, smallpox, typhoid fever, the flu. But the worst was yellow fever.

Doctor Gordon knew his dance with the captain was about to begin, particularly on a ship with the *Franklin's* reputation. He had to assume the captain and crew had worked hard to ready the ship for the inspection.

A cool but humid breeze out of the southwest flowed from Portsmouth's tidal marshes and over the ship's deck as the skipper strode out to meet Gordon. The doctor got straight to the point.

"Has there been any sickness on board?"

"None," Byram said. "Both the passengers and the crew have been perfectly healthy for the ten-day voyage."

"Everyone? Every single crew and passenger?"

"Well," Byram admitted, "I lost two men, the first a fireman who died suddenly, I supposed from a heart attack, for he had been well and at work a short time before his death. He had been taken suddenly with sharp pain in the left side, and great difficulty of breathing, and died in half an hour after his seizure."[17]

The second man, Byram explained, had taken the place of the first, shoveling coal into the ship's furnaces. He wasn't used to the heat and the strenuous work and died of exhaustion. Neither showed symptoms of yellow fever, the captain said.

Gordon inspected the ship and found it clean. The crew, at least the few he could find to speak with, seemed healthy. Byram didn't disclose the cases on his ship in Saint Thomas, and he'd lied about the cause of the two deaths. He left out that his passengers had been so desperate to get off the *Franklin* that they risked death to change ships in open water. He failed to mention the boy they'd buried at sea.

Gordon knew yellow fever had been rampant in Saint Thomas that spring. Ships that arrived in March and April had told him as much, so it was odd when Byram didn't mention the epidemic on the island. Byram begged Gordon to allow him to come into port and used one true story to support his case. The *Franklin* was in desperate need of repair, still leaking so steadily that the crew was continuously pumping out water to keep her afloat. Byram begged to slip into one of Portsmouth's shipyards, get the leaks patched, and be on his way.

The doctor sympathized, but the captain's desperation made him wary. He ordered the *Franklin* to stay anchored at quarantine. He'd give it a few more days to see if anything broke out on board. Gordon could tell that the long days at sea had taken a toll on the captain. It would be fine if the crew went into the cities for a meal and some civilization, he said.

Gordon was like the rest of the people in the coastal ports: He knew the "symptoms" he was looking for—sick crew, deaths—but not the cause or what conditions might foment an epidemic. The people in these cities only knew that disease typically came on a week or so after a heavy rain and ended in the fall with the first hard frost. They knew it came aboard ships but wrongly thought that it spread through the air in stinky gases that floated up from the marshes or the stale air trapped in a ship's hold. They even had a name for what they thought caused the fever, headache, and chills: "bad air," otherwise known as "mal-air-ia."

A few years earlier, Alabama surgeon Doctor Josiah Clark Nott had become the first to suggest that mosquitoes transmitted yellow fever. It made no sense, Nott said, that a vapor or gas emitted by a ship, a marsh, or a pile of rotting garbage would be swept along by the breeze and spread a virus. "We can well understand how insects wafted by the winds (as happens with mosquitoes, flying ants, many of the Aphides, etc.) should haul up on the first tree, house or other object in their course, offering a resting place." But Nott's observation could not be proved, and no one heeded it. The goal remained to stop ships from importing bad air.[18]

The local papers logged the ships that came into port, noting which ones were ordered to fly yellow flags. It was a big deal but a frequent one, so even with the *Franklin* at anchorage, Norfolk and Portsmouth residents went about their business. That spring, the cities were blossoming into their usual flurry of daily life, with church bells announcing each hour and horses and wagons clattering down cobblestone streets and echoing off the narrowly clustered houses like drumbeats. Hammering and sawing noises emanated from the shipyards and skipped across the Elizabeth River. Gulls swooped and shrieked.

The river was the spine between Norfolk and Portsmouth, and ferries, steamers, fishermen, and shipyard workers plied those waters day and night. The *Franklin* sat in quarantine at the point that was essentially the head on the spine, and people on either shore could see at least a silhouette of whatever went on across that wide, calm harbor.

On the Norfolk shore directly across from the *Franklin*, a man named William Harper and a crew worked every day to repair a Revolutionary War station called Fort Norfolk. As they worked, they warily watched the activity on the ship's deck. After seeing a current of decaying oranges and bananas floating in the river, Harper and others paddled out to the *Franklin*, ostensibly to see if they could get some fruit before it all rotted.

"We'd like to speak to the first mate," Harper asked as they arrived. "He's down with the fever."

Harper learned that the first mate wasn't the only one sick, and that was all he needed to hear.[19] He and the men nearly ran off the deck, paddled back to shore, and became obsessed with watching for any curious movement on the ship. It didn't take long. A few days later, they saw men laboring to drag a rolled mattress onto the deck, remove a corpse, and put it into a box. They watched as the crew flung the mattress overboard, then moved to the far side of the ship. Harper spotted a dinghy rowing toward the Portsmouth shore. By then, more than rotten fruit was washing up at the fort. First came a mattress, then a man's body. The dead man was dressed as a coal heaver, or fireman, from a ship. His face was mutilated, which Harper and his crew figured had likely happened in the river after he had died. The corpse had one more, gravely disturbing, characteristic: His hands were as yellow as lemons.

A few evenings later, Harper's crew watched as two men came onto the deck at dusk, scurried one way and then another, then glanced around. They raced toward the railing, then climbed over it. Both hesitated. *Surely, they wouldn't,* Harper must have thought. No sane person would jump into the Elizabeth River; the cities built on opposite sides of the river had been making efforts to improve their cleanliness—by sloping the streets to drain downhill. All the garbage, horse manure, animal entrails, rotten food, and fetid ballast water from ships slid downhill into the river. The salty water stunk like a pasture.

The men shinnied down the wooden sides of the *Franklin* and jumped in.[20]

Harper and his crew dropped their shovels and hurried over to the river's edge. They watched as one man's head popped up. His arms flailed as he treaded water to locate the shore, then he started swimming. They couldn't see the second man. At last, a second silhouette bobbed above the surface, and both flailed their way toward the fort. Harper and the crew swung into action.

For protection against the British, the military had built Fort Norfolk behind a high berm and seawall that swimmers couldn't breach. As the men from the *Franklin* neared the shore, Harper's crew threw ropes over to them and winched them onto the berm. They lay gasping. The crew stood in quiet shock, then one spoke up.

"Why did you risk your lives like that?"

"Better to chance drowning," one said, wheezing for air, "than stay on the ship and face certain death."[21]

William Harper's reputation for honesty was sterling, and what happened at the fort was one more thing Gordon surely related when conferring with the Norfolk Board of Health and several members of the Portsmouth Common Council. The cities hadn't had a serious outbreak of the fever in three decades, a fact they touted regularly. But they couldn't stop damaged ships from coming into the harbor to get worked on.

The city boards detailed their concerns, then put it all back on Gordon: Lay your eyes on the *Franklin*, walk every inch of it, then you make the call. On Tuesday, June 19, Gordon boarded the ship for a second time. Byram met him on deck. The crew members who weren't sick and hadn't escaped had spent days scrubbing and polishing the *Franklin* to prepare for the inspection. Byram took Gordon below deck, to the engine room and into the ship's hold. The only ballast was some salted ham—and ten thirty-two-pound iron cannons.

Gordon asked Byram if he had arranged for repairs at a specific shipyard.

"Yes, Page and Allen's in Gosport."

Page and Allen's was a small business, squeezed next to the massive Navy Yard where fifteen hundred men toiled every day. Hundreds of Irish laborers and their extended families lived in cramped and shoddily built apartments within a short walk of where the *Franklin* would dock. The swampy streets, combined with decaying wood in the marshes and old piers, would serve as a massive petri dish.

The fact was, though, Byram had done everything that was asked of him. The hold where everyone believed the disease fomented looked clean. Gordon couldn't find a reason to keep the *Franklin* at quarantine.

"You may go to Page and Allen's," Gordon told the captain, "but there is one condition. Under no circumstances can you break out and empty the cargo hold."[22]

Gordon climbed off the ship.

Within minutes, the *Franklin* lifted anchor and sailed into the heart of the cities.

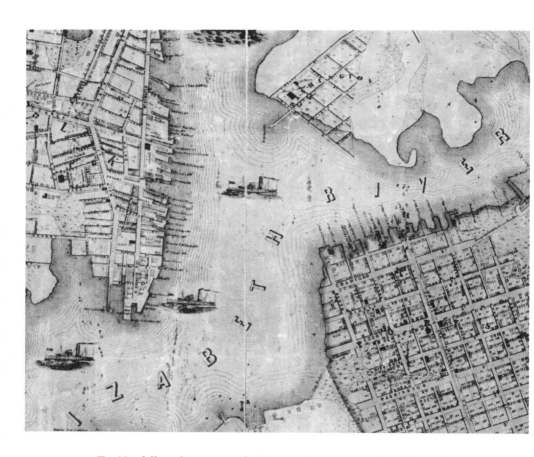

The Norfolk and Portsmouth, Virginia, harbor, with Norfolk on the left, from James Keily's 1851 *Map of the city of Norfolk and the town of Portsmouth*, Library of Congress.

CHAPTER TWO
CITIES ON THE RISE

B Y 1855, it seemed to everyone that Norfolk's destiny was to become the New York of the South. Government leaders, as well as historians and newspaper pundits, were perplexed that the city wasn't already among the most vibrant in the country—with good reason. A bird's-eye view of Norfolk and Portsmouth shows a stunningly lucky perch on the Atlantic Coast. The cities rest on part of the Eastern Seaboard just above where North Carolina juts into the ocean, like an awning protecting them from the worst Atlantic storms. The Virginia port sits halfway up the coast, six-hundred-odd miles north of Florida, six-hundred-odd miles south of Portland, Maine.

Virginia's far southeast corner boasts a moderate climate compared with competing port cities like New York and Boston, so the river rarely ices over. Its harbor features uncommonly deep water and is nestled tight with land all around to buffer the winds. Just downriver, three of the country's most critical bodies of water swirl together: the Atlantic Ocean, the Chesapeake Bay, and the James River. Norfolk and Portsmouth have always had a nearly unfair advantage over their port city competition.

In the 1800s, most ships sailed up the coast from the West Indies, then steered westward into the confluence of the Chesapeake Bay and

James River, where the British first came ashore in 1607. From there, a mariner would navigate due south and coast into the calm waters of the Elizabeth River. The harbor lay snuggled between the shipbuilding and repair yards of Portsmouth on its south bank and the two dozen commercial wharves of Norfolk on its north.[23]

Thomas Jefferson, who had no desire to live in Norfolk partly due to its aggressive mosquitoes, nonetheless saw the city's potential to dominate shipping from its strategic spot in the middle of the Atlantic Seaboard. Norfolk, Jefferson predicted, would become "the great Emporium of the Chesapeake."

Half a century later, in 1851, a London correspondent of a New York newspaper noted that steamships would soon be built to haul ten thousand tons of cargo and one thousand passengers across the Atlantic from the new world to the old in six days. Ships of that size and that amount of cargo would require deep harbors. "Neither New York nor Liverpool has sufficient water in their channels to meet the views that are now in embryo," the correspondent wrote. Norfolk, with its sixty-foot-deep harbor, would become one of the great ports of the United States, he predicted.

President Millard Fillmore, also during a visit to the city that same year, talked of Norfolk's nearly ideal position and its naturally deep and protected harbor. "It's surprising that the common port of Norfolk and Portsmouth had not been chosen as the site of a New York instead of that city. I cannot divest myself of the belief that the time is not distant when Norfolk will rival the proudest cities of the Union."[24]

The city had developed a bustle. In 1850, Norfolk's gas works opened and first lit Freemason Street, then the rest of downtown; glowing silver lights swept along streets in a checkerboard pattern. Mariners entering the harbor could see the city dotted with elegant warm lights. The city established Norfolk Military Academy for boys and Norfolk Female Institute for girls. In 1845, when Norfolk officially became a city, it erected a grand, new City Hall. The architect for the dome was Thomas Ustick Walter, who had designed the dome of the US Capitol and its separate wings for the Senate and the House.

As evidence of the depth of the Virginia harbor and its strategic importance to the country, the USS *Pennsylvania* steamed directly from the Philadelphia shipyard, where it was built, to the Gosport Navy Yard to make its home at the river's edge in Portsmouth. The Navy Yard, just across the Elizabeth River from Norfolk, had built the nation's first dry dock where ships could be hoisted out of the water for repair, a suitable place to house the nation's largest warship. More than fifteen hundred men hammered and sawed every day, building or fixing ships just a couple of hundred yards down the street from where the *Benjamin Franklin* was tied up to the pier.

Though not as glamorous as gaslit streets, Norfolk had vastly improved its sanitation in the decade leading up to 1855. Starting in the mid-1840s, cholera leapfrogged around the world's cities, including Norfolk in 1849. An infamous cholera outbreak in London in 1854 spread through contamination of a public well. Doctor John Snow marked cholera deaths on a street-by-street map and pinpointed the center of the spread. He walked to the midpoint of the largest cluster of deaths, found a public well pump, and removed the handle. The outbreak stopped.[25]

To assure safe drinking water, Norfolk leaders had earlier considered building a water tower twenty miles away at Deep Creek, then piping the water into the city, or hauling fifteen hundred barrels of water at a time on a steamboat into a reservoir near downtown. Residents grew tired of waiting and built private cisterns, which they considered to be a reliable source of drinking water, right next to their homes.

Cisterns were brick reservoirs built into the ground, filling rainwater through pipes that channeled the water from the eaves of the house and the gutters. One problem residents were unaware of: The cisterns offered an attractive breeding spot for mosquitoes—fresh still water within a short flight of the people they fed on.

Two years earlier, thirty-six-year-old historian William S. Forrest published a five-hundred-seven-page book with the deceptively dull title *Historical and Descriptive Sketches of Norfolk and Vicinity*. He unleashed multiple punches at the men who were holding the city back. He was the perfect messenger for the task. Forrest had founded a newspaper, the *Virginia Temperance Advocate*, dedicated to temperance, morality, literature, and health. A century later, Norfolk history columnist George H. Tucker assessed that Forrest had been "blessed with a knack of never forgetting intimate details concerning persons and important happenings."[26]

Now, Forrest and the progressive thinkers in Norfolk and Portsmouth were miffed at the slow pace of development.

"When the peculiar and natural advantages of Norfolk, and of the sister town on the opposite side of the river, are considered, it must be admitted by all that these places should long have been numbered among the great cities of the Union."

Unlike casual observers, Forrest was not the least bit perplexed about why Norfolk had underachieved, and the reason had a name: the Virginia legislature. When the era of ocean steamships began in the late 1830s, Great Britain took the lead and built a paddle-propelled steamship that crossed the Atlantic in sixteen days. France would have none of that, and it sought to compete with a transatlantic steamship line sailing into and out of Norfolk.

The Virginia legislature voted down France's proposal for the steamship line, and the transatlantic route was instead established in Boston.

"If the charter would have been granted, Norfolk would have been the center of steam navigation in the United States," Forrest said. "The lines to the Isthmus (Panama before a canal) would have belonged to Norfolk, and probably, the lines to Havre (France) and Bremen (Germany). But Boston got the line of steamers, sent its ship to Liverpool, and recovered all the trade."

Forrest blamed the former policy of Great Britain in blocking shipping channels off the Virginia coast, the state legislature's refusal to fund the port's growth, and older residents who "have appeared to be satisfied with slow and gradual progress." Some still were dead set against "nearly every innovation," but by 1853, Forrest saw a tendril of hope that a more enterprising attitude pervaded most of the public. Though not booming as quickly as Forrest and others wished, the cities were growing.

Norfolk now had five fire companies, desperately needed due to all the wooden structures. It had a US District Court, a Customs House, eight banks, five daily newspapers, and a humane society for helping the poor. Steamship lines connected Norfolk and Portsmouth to other Atlantic Coast cities, running to New York and Philadelphia once a week, Richmond three times a week, Washington, DC, twice a week, and up the Chesapeake Bay to Baltimore every day.[27]

But Virginia cities lagged far behind their trading partners in rail connections. Forrest and others saw this as both a great injustice of the past decade and something with terrific potential. Though it was a baby step, Norfolk and Portsmouth together established the Seaboard and Roanoke Railroad company, linking downtown Portsmouth to Weldon, North Carolina. It was one thing to have steamship routes tying together port cities, but the upstart country, its people and trade, now reached toward the vast open West. Norfolk had already lost numerous residents, the risk-taking entrepreneurial types, who left in 1849 to join the rush for gold in California.

A transcontinental railroad was a wisp of an idea, and the leaders of the Seaboard and Roanoke Railroad—named for its end point on the Roanoke River—wanted to stitch their line together with other railroads to reach the Mississippi River. The Seaboard and Roanoke's eighty-five-mile track would fuse with a second railroad to get to Raleigh, another to get to Knoxville, Tennessee, then another to Chattanooga, and yet another to cross Tennessee to Memphis. In all, some seven railroads would haul people and goods nine-hundred-eight miles from Memphis to Norfolk, which could then ship them anywhere in the world.

"When these railroads are completed, the rush of produce down them from the Mississippi to this point of the Atlantic seaboard must be immense," Forrest wrote.

At last, maybe the Virginia port would assume its rightful place as one of the country's critical commercial hubs, Forrest hoped.

By the summer of 1855, though, political rumblings flipped the country on its head.

EVEN BEFORE THE infamous potato famine, America had always been a magnet for the Irish. Few seemed alarmed in the 1700s when mostly Presbyterians from the northern part of Ireland arrived in Boston, Philadelphia, and New York, or that a quarter million Irish lived in the country by the time the Revolutionary War broke out.

Then the Catholics came. These immigrants from farther south in Ireland arrived in waves during the first half of the 1800s, nearly a million landing in America from 1820 to 1845. American contractors took out advertisements in Dublin newspapers to man such big construction projects as the Erie Canal. With pickaxes and shovels, Irish men working for a dollar a day dug that 363-mile canal.

In Virginia in the 1850s, eight hundred Irish workers along with forty enslaved Africans dug through the Blue Ridge Mountains at Rockfish Gap, chiseling, blasting, and pickaxing out a 4,237-foot rail tunnel for the Blue Ridge Railroad. The workers' wives and children stayed with them, living in makeshift camps along the unfinished railroad bed. Nearly two hundred men, women, and children died during the dig through the mountain, many from a cholera epidemic.[28]

At home, the Irish had toiled as tenant farmers for English and Irish Protestants who had confiscated their land and become overlord barons.[29] The British government acknowledged that half of Irish families in the countryside lived in one-room mud cabins without chimneys for heat. Many slept on straw on the dirt floor, which they often shared with the family's pigs and chickens.

But the Irish had one thing that most impoverished people did not: potatoes. More than three million Irish lived almost exclusively off potatoes, packed with nutrients like carbohydrates, protein, vitamin C, B6, and potassium. For many years, Ireland's extremely poor were better nourished than the English underclass, which subsisted mostly on bread. But that changed, too, in 1845. That autumn, the leaves on potato plants turned black, shriveled, then rotted. Many thought a fog over the region caused the blight, and they weren't too far off. An airborne fungus had crept in on ships steaming from North America to Southern England, then wafted across the Irish Sea.[30]

In previous decades, the Irish had survived multiple bad harvest years, but none that gripped the entire country at once. They rationed their way through the winter of 1845, able to do so because about half of the potato crop was edible and by selling off their livestock. They figured if only they could muddle on until the next harvest, they'd be okay. They had never seen crops fail in two consecutive years.

But the black blight stayed for the next four years as their English rulers sat and watched. They adhered to a popular theory of the day called laissez-faire, which translated to do nothing and see what happens. The English never, during the famine, provided widespread food shipments to the Irish over fear it would make food prices in England jump. In fact, even with the Irish dying of starvation, the English maintained their tight grip on exports and shipped massive amounts of wheat, barley, and oatmeal out of Ireland.

So, the Irish fled. They boarded ships with almost nothing to their names and came to North America by the hundreds of thousands. In one case, in June 1847, a medical inspection station in Quebec harbor became overwhelmed. Forty ships hauling fourteen thousand Irish immigrants waited for health checks in a line that stretched two miles down the Saint Lawrence River.[31]

In New York alone, six hundred fifty thousand Irish arrived during the famine years. From the moment they stepped off boats, they were harassed and conned out of whatever paltry funds they had. "Runners," who seemed friendly because they spoke Gaelic, found the newcomers and directed them to boarding houses they touted as having warm meals, storage for their belongings, and cheap rent in a clean place. They'd arrive and find a boarding house teeming with rodents, costing four times what was promised, and were jammed into rooms with ten other wide-eyed Irish. When their money ran out, they were kicked out and their belongings sold to cover the back rent.[32]

In Boston, as elsewhere in the country, building codes, fire and safety codes, and sanitary laws didn't exist. Landlords could do whatever they wanted. Homeowners chopped up waterfront mansions, formerly occupied by well-off merchants, into small rooms that crammed one hundred Irish into a single house.

In the 1840s, nearly eight hundred thousand Irish immigrated to America. In the next decade, nine hundred fourteen thousand more arrived. There were now more Irish in New York City than in Dublin, and they made up 43 percent of the foreign-born population across the country.[33]

Because of their sheer numbers, their poverty, and the fact that they had lived in close quarters with extended family back home, most of the Irish Catholic immigrants settled in cities. There were simply too many of them for all to end up in New York, Boston, or Philadelphia, so they surged into Albany, Chicago, Pittsburgh, even Butte, Montana. They rolled into Baltimore, Savannah, and Charleston, South Carolina, and, of course, into Norfolk and Portsmouth.

In Norfolk, the new arrivals packed into rows of tenements crammed onto filled marshland called Barry's Row. Over in Portsmouth, they flocked to a burg called Gosport, where twice a day the tide crept up to the back of the tenements, often flowing into their basements.

Locals called those hastily built, and never maintained, tenements "Leigh's Row," or just "Irish Row," where as many as six hundred Irish men, women, and children lived in just a few dozen apartments. The men worked at the Gosport Navy Yard or one of the even closer small ship repair yards that they could see from their tenements.

One of them was Page and Allen's Shipyard, where the *Franklin* docked for repairs.

IF FOR EVERY action there is an equal and opposite reaction, the deluge of Irish into America spawned a rapid reflex of hatred and discrimination. The waves of Irish landing in American cities meant that, very soon, Catholicism would be the majority Christian denomination in the country. The thinking went that Irish Catholics would have more allegiance to the pope than their new country's laws and leaders, and that couldn't be allowed to happen.

In Boston, Protestant workers torched a convent. In Philadelphia, Protestant mobs attacked groups of Irish, who retaliated. Gangs of the two sects waged brutal street fights for three days.[34] In New York, an archbishop heard of the Philadelphia attacks and sent armed Irishmen to stand guard at the Catholic churches. He then went to New York's mayor with a stern warning: If one Catholic church was touched, he'd dispatch Irish to set ablaze all of Manhattan. Anti-Irish sentiment became in vogue. In many cities, where most of the Irish had settled, newspaper ads listed available apartments and jobs with the tagline "Positively No Irish Need Apply." Handbills posted around Boston read, "All Catholics and all persons who favor the Catholic Church are vile imposters, liars, villains, and cowardly cutthroats."[35]

Out of the stench of this steaming pile of resentment arose an underground fraternity known as the Order of the Star Spangled Banner. Emerging in New York in 1850, the Order had secret passwords and hand signs, an initiation rite, and a requirement that members prove they were pure-blooded Anglo-Saxon Protestants. They recruited members quietly, a few at a time, and organized in local groups called "Councils" or "Lodges." Then they transformed into a political organization, called the American Party, a third party to take on the Whigs and Democrats.

The American Party stood for deporting poverty-stricken immigrants, a twenty-one-year waiting period for new arrivals to become citizens, mandatory Bible reading in schools, and the elimination of all Catholics from political office. American Party supporters were to keep their membership secret. If anyone asked if they were involved, they were to respond, "I know nothing." Soon, the American Party simply became "The Know Nothings."

Propelled by Irish hatred in Boston, Know Nothings dominated the spring 1854 elections for the state legislature in Massachusetts. In Philadelphia, the Whig candidate for mayor, Robert T. Conrad, let it be known during his campaign that he was clandestinely a Know Nothing, promising to close bars on Sundays and appoint only native-born Americans to office. He romped to victory. In Washington, DC, a Know Nothing candidate defeated the incumbent mayor.

The momentum that winning brings, the panic it puts into the other party, and the hope it brings to supporters now powered the Know Nothings. So far, they had only flexed their political power up North, but they planned to fix that with an offensive in the Virginia election for governor in May 1855. They'd run candidates for state legislature and City Councils as well.

The nation's eyes would be on the Virginia races since the state was the largest in the South and elected its governor the year before the presidential campaign. This time, Norfolk and Portsmouth would be front and center in the battle. If the Know Nothings could make a stand in Virginia, the bellwether of the South, they'd truly have a national party. It seemed like they already had cells of operation throughout the Old Dominion.

Millard Fillmore, president of the country from 1850 to 1853 as a member of the Whig party, had his eye on the Virginia election. He hoped to ride the Know Nothing wave back into the White House in 1856. Solomon G. Haven, a Whig congressman from New York, paid a quiet visit to Virginia and reported back to Fillmore, "There is hardly a schoolhouse or cross-roads or blacksmith's shop but the boys have an organization there."[36]

In November 1854, the pro-slavery Democrats met in Staunton, Virginia, for a nomination convention. Former Congressman Henry A. Wise, who was unliked by state Democratic leaders, showed up with a twelve-thousand-word screed in which each sentence landed body blows against the Know Nothing doctrine. Wise was the guy who would swing the cudgel like the Democrats needed. He took the nomination and immediately set out to get the word to as many parts of the state as he could. No group of voters was too small for Wise. Virginians had rarely seen a politician with such conviction and vigor.

In the language of the day, Wise called out members of the Order as hypocrites: "The (Know Nothing) party's indictment against the Papacy recites its own crimes against humanity. The Church of Rome was never more intolerant than this treacherous champion of liberty."

Wise had another ace in his pocket. The Know Nothings had emerged from a movement in Massachusetts, and the men at the center of that were abolitionists. Though Southern Know Nothings remained pro-slavery, editors of Democratic party newspapers constantly seeded the idea that once in office the party would abolish it. In January 1855, the *Daily Richmond Enquirer* claimed that the unspoken intent of the Know Nothings was "to strike down the institutions of the South."

As Wise traveled the state bloodying the Know Nothing ideology, the Know Nothings disappeared behind a curtain of secrecy. For an election held in late May, they didn't even nominate a candidate until March. At long last, the Know Nothings' convention drew a crowd of former Whigs and Democrats, and they nominated Thomas Flournoy, a fiery activist and former Whig who they hoped had the credibility to attract former Whigs to the polls. The Know Nothing plan for the issue of slavery was simple: They wouldn't discuss it.[37]

Flournoy thought he had the election in the bag. He figured that when the polls opened, members of the secret Know Nothing lodges would pop out of those blacksmith shops, crossroads, and schoolhouses and sweep him to victory. A story circulated in Whig newspapers, which were converting quickly to Know Nothing papers, that gave them hope.

Wise was at a campaign barbecue in April, hammering Know Nothing supporters. Their secrecy was really cowardice, a lack of honor, a scar on their manliness.

I wonder if there is a single Know Nothing brave enough, confident enough in his beliefs, to declare them here today? Wise asked.

No one in the room spoke.

I challenge any Know Nothing to take the stage and debate me, Wise said.

The room was again quiet. Wise waited in silence to allow the cowardice to sink in. Finally, an older man in the back stood. Wise nodded toward him. The man turned, not toward Wise but to face the crowd. He called out, "SAM, STAND UP!"[38]

Know Nothings had nicknamed their party "Sam," a character they'd created to represent Uncle Sam's nephew. And stand they did. Two of every three men in the room stood to confront Wise. Flabbergasted, Wise walked off.

Flournoy's campaign reflected the Know Nothing's cockiness. After receiving the nomination, he wrote an acceptance letter. Then he went to his home in Halifax County and sat on his front porch.[39]

In May, Wise stomped Flournoy by ten thousand votes. Flournoy's vote count would have won any previous statewide election in Virginia, but turbulent topics of slavery and immigration had drawn the most voters ever.

Slavery would remain a Virginia institution if the governor of the South's most populous state had a say. But the Know Nothings had not been vanquished. They'd won the seats for the mayor of Chicago, and the governors of Maryland, Rhode Island, and California. Senators

Sam Houston of Texas and Anthony Kennedy of Maryland became Know Nothings, as did Samuel Morse, who invented the telegraph and Morse code, and Henry Wilson, the eighteenth vice president of the United States.

The Know Nothings remained a force in Virginia, especially in urban areas. They were voted onto councils in Fairfax, Parkersburg (now in West Virginia), and in Alexandria, where the Know Nothing mayoral candidate crushed his Democrat opponent.

Those who read the *New York Times* on June 28, 1855, learned of Know Nothing dominance in Norfolk: "Full returns of our municipal election show the success of the entire American ticket, except the Mayor and Gauger of Liquors."

The results of the mayor's race flummoxed many. Thirty-three-year-old attorney Hunter Woodis had taken the seat. He was a clever, likable man who seemed to stand for everyone, regardless of where they were born. And he was Irish Catholic.

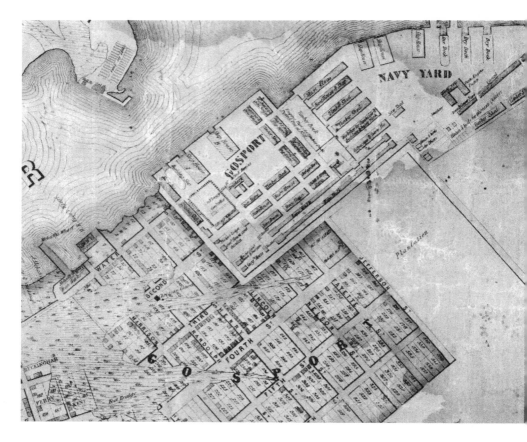

A view of Gosport, with Page and Allen's Shipyard on the left, from James Kelly's 1851 map.

CHAPTER THREE
OUTBREAK

THE *Franklin* crew had barely lashed the ship to the wharf that June 19 when Captain Byram did everything the port's health officer told him not to do. He pumped fetid ballast water onto the soggy pier, then told the shipyard workers where the problem was, down in the hold. They lowered themselves into the belly of the ship and began to work on the engines and boilers.[40]

Days passed, though, and no one got sick.

About a week later, Doctor Joseph Schoolfield got word that a woman named Martha Fox, who lived about a mile outside town, was stricken with perplexing symptoms. Schoolfield made his way to her house, situated on a point where fingers of salt water intruded on the land then retreated. Creeks and marshes enveloped it on three sides, too. Fox could see the wide part of the Elizabeth River from there. She could smell the salt air and watch herons spear crabs in the shallow waters. From her upper-floor windows, she could see the *Franklin* sitting in quarantine.[41]

Schoolfield wouldn't have been summoned unless her symptoms were severe. As a member of Portsmouth's Sanitary Committee, his senses were always attuned not just to his patients but for cases that could be a harbinger of a festering fever, cholera, typhoid—anything that could mushroom and inflict the whole town. Schoolfield knew the Fox house well. He'd visited a couple of years earlier when Fox's daughter had taken ill. The house was on what locals called a "garden farm," land devoted entirely to growing fruits and vegetables. Schoolfield, and many others, believed the stench from rotting food, decomposing animals, or even the air of marshes themselves could spawn yellow fever.

"At that time all around the house the ground was covered with decaying vegetable matter, particularly cucumbers, of which many thousands were rotting on the vines within a stone's throw of her window," the doctor noted in his log of the visit.

Schoolfield logged that the ground was spongy that morning, his boots going squish-squash, squish-squash as he walked to the house. The previous afternoon, thunder squalls had dumped more than half an inch of rain.[42] Martha Fox had moved down to Portsmouth from New Jersey just six weeks earlier to join her son and grandchildren. The doctor knew that someone who lived outside of town, near a marsh, coming down with a summer fever was a fairly typical occurrence.

When Schoolfield went inside and saw Fox, he immediately figured her condition indicated a typical case of bilious fever—an elevated body temperature, accompanied by nausea, vomiting, or diarrhea. A determination of bilious fever, though, wasn't technically a diagnosis of the root cause—it was more a broad description of symptoms.[43]

"She complained greatly of pain in her head," Schoolfield wrote in his log. "The skin was hot and dry, and the thirst great. The tongue was large and flabby and covered with a thick fur. The eyes were red and injected."

She kept demanding ice and water, but she threw up immediately after drinking. She was so restless that her family could barely keep her in bed.

Fox's symptoms baffled Schoolfield. On one hand, he figured, she was likely more susceptible than most to an attack, being an "old lady" at the age of sixty-three. And she likely suffered more than most would due to her recent arrival and lack of acclimation to the South's warmer weather. But she was the only case in the neighborhood. No one else in the family was sick. She hadn't been to town since arriving, so there was little chance she'd picked up something contagious.

Fox's fever retreated after a few days, but her nausea and vomiting worsened. She began throwing up dark matter. After a few more days, her brain shut down and she went into a deep stupor.

"After death," Schoolfield logged, "the peculiar lemon tinge of skin, so characteristic of yellow fever, was very distinct."

Schoolfield's thoughts now jumped to the *Franklin*. As part of the Sanitary Committee, he knew where the ship had been each day, anchored in quarantine within sight of the Fox house. But he saw little possibility of that causing the fever.

"It would hardly be contended that the malaria was carried so far through the air in potency sufficient to generate the fever. To have reached her residence, the wind must have blown from the north-east, and there were only two days in June in which it came from that quarter—some seven or eight days before Mrs. Fox was attacked."[44]

He didn't yet know, in fact few people did, that crew members from the *Franklin* had ferried their dead shipmate's body and buried him on the side of the river near Fox's house.

Either way, Schoolfield kept his thinking to himself. He couldn't prove anything. Based on the facts, and his understanding of the cause and spread of yellow fever, the link he needed to connect Fox's death back to the *Franklin* didn't exist. But that possibility would continue to gnaw at him as the days passed.

As for the rest of the town's residents, hardly anyone knew Fox, so word of her death didn't spread quickly or far. Schoolfield figured that Portsmouth had nothing to be concerned about unless things moved closer to the main part of town. Then, they did.

A week and a half after the *Franklin* docked at Page and Allen's Shipyard, Doctor John Trugien was summoned to a house on Water Street, just about one hundred feet from the ship in Gosport.

Trugien was twenty-eight years old and full of energy and passion for practicing medicine in his hometown. He'd grown up poor yet clearly had a wealth of intelligence. He spent most of his youth reading whatever he could find. When he turned eighteen, his parents couldn't afford to send him to college. Instead, they arranged an apprenticeship with Schoolfield. After four years of seeing just about any sickness or injury that came through the door, he studied for two years at the University of Maryland, then trained at the University of Pennsylvania in Philadelphia, the nation's first medical school.[45] His classmates explored the health problems that crippled cities and perplexed doctors: typhoid fever, pneumonia, scarlet fever, the treatment of bilious remittent fever, and marsh miasma. Trugien's dissertation did not address the individual health issues of the day and instead revealed the kind of broad curiosity he could bring to medical care: He researched the "human eye."

Just two years out of medical school, he got one of his cases—about a man who was stabbed and lived for five days until he stood to walk against doctors' orders—published in the prestigious *American Journal of Medical Science*. His sincerity and enthusiasm, along with his mission to bring modern, big-city medicine to his small hometown brought him trust with his patients. Within a couple of years, Trugien had a sterling reputation and had built one of the larger practices in Portsmouth.

It was already hot that Saturday morning, June 30. The thermometer had hit ninety-six the day before, and the skies bore a fuzzy-hazy blue as the temperature headed for at least ninety-two degrees. Trugien made his way from the main part of Portsmouth over to Gosport.

Portsmouth was an old town, made official before the Revolutionary War, its High Street twice as wide as its other streets, sufficient for carriages to pass without trouble and with room for people walking and vegetable farmers hawking their produce. It was wide enough, in fact, for the tracks for the new Seaboard and Roanoke

Railroad, which screeched and billowed smoke down the right side of
the street to its wharf on the Elizabeth River. The street was lined on
each side with rows of two- or three-story drug stores, grocers, banks,
hardware stores, and even taller churches and hotels. Colorful, stately
homes, in the style now being built during Queen Victoria's reign in
England, framed the streets. How far residences extended on either
side of High Street depended on where solid ground ended and tidal
marsh infiltrated and made building impossible.[46] Unlike Norfolk's
streets, Portsmouth's were not paved or drained but remained solid
dirt, until it rained.

About ten thousand people lived in Portsmouth, with at least
twenty-five hundred being either freed Blacks or the enslaved.

Gosport was technically part of Portsmouth, though it was very
much another world, accessed by one main route. That morning,
Trugien would have made his way down Crawford Street, which ran
north-south a block back and parallel to the Elizabeth River. From the
Crawford Hotel at the corner of High Street, he passed J.K. Cooke's
Steam Saw Mill at the edge of a vast marsh and stepped onto an earthen
bridge. The causeway—eight hundred feet long and twenty feet
across—was covered in layer after layer of wood chips from the nearby
shipbuilding yards yet was barely usable in wet weather or for many
days after a hard rain. Trugien could hear the swamp mud gurgling
and popping as tiny marsh crabs scurried around, then ducked into
mud tunnels to avoid the screeching gulls and slow-stalking herons.

Baking in the summer sun, the marsh reeked. All the streets
drained into the marshes, so they were "receptacles of all the filth of
the town. On their margins, in many places, are pig-pens, stables and
other nuisances."[47]

For most Portsmouth residents, the town ended at the causeway.
A resident of the main part of Portsmouth would not cross that bridge
unless he or she had a reason.

Gosport was essentially a company town for shipbuilding and
repair. The first business across the bridge was Mehaffy's Wharf,

containing Gosport Iron Works. The street dead-ended three blocks later at the massive Gosport Navy Yard, one of the largest Navy yards in the country. It stretched across nearly three thousand feet of shoreline, with three massive dry docks, three ship houses, eight timber sheds, a saw shed, sheds for riggings and sails, and an iron storehouse. The shipyard commander lived on the property, in a classic house and garden, with just slightly smaller houses and yards for other officers and their families.

The shipyard had been around since 1767, making it the country's oldest Navy repair yard. Its entrance, on the inland side of town, was an architectural masterpiece: It covered a third of the width of the entire yard, a three-story building with fourteen dormers above windows on the left side, fourteen dormers with windows on the right, and a gateway entrance in the middle with four classical columns and a cupola and bell tower on the top.

Much of the ground beneath the Navy Yard buildings was known as "made land." In the 1800s, people feared that what emanated from swamps created "mal-air-ia," or bad air, so port cities turned water into land to improve air quality. The Navy had dumped the mud dug out for the yard's docks, dredged out sludge from the river bottom, and dumped bark, wood chips, shavings, even boards from old sheds and boats into the low-lying wetland on the property. They graded that land so it would drain, then built on top of it.

Crawford Street became Water Street on the Gosport side of the causeway, and two blocks short of the Navy Yard sat Page and Allen's Shipyard. Though a small yard, Page and Allen's was well-known: Two years earlier, it had built a ship named *Neptune's Car*, a two-hundred-sixteen-foot clipper designed for the speed needed to get from New York to San Francisco around Cape Horn. The rush for gold in California was on, creating demand for the rapid transportation of food and supplies. Earlier that year, *Neptune's Car* had made the fourteen-thousand-mile sail in one hundred and one days. She would become known as the only clipper ship built in the South.[48]

On his house call, Trugien would have noticed the long ship, the *Benjamin Franklin*, docked at the yard and heard the echoes of hammering from those working on repairs.

As a Portsmouth native, he knew that Page and Allen's wharf had been there long before the shipyard. Years ago, it had been a hub of foreign trade, primarily for imports from the West Indies. The pine logs that formed the old wharf were rotting and their "pores saturated with water."[49]

The wharf was covered several inches thick with wood chips and shavings from ship building, an attempt to keep it usable and dry. At the end, a three-story-tall brick warehouse ran parallel to the river. A thirty- to forty-foot-wide dock skirted the landside edge of the warehouse, the dock again covered with refuse from the shipyard to keep it solid."

"In this way an extensive mass of woody matter, several feet deep, has been formed, upon which the rain and river water, and the burning rays of a southern sun are constantly acting," Schoolfield described in a report later that summer.

At the rear of that same block just a hundred or so feet away, fronting Water Street, stood a row of eight three-story brick apartment buildings. They were built in the past few years to house the Irish who had been drawn to Portsmouth by the promise of work in the shipyards. Schoolfield couldn't hide his disgust for this part of town and had no empathy for the Irish workers and their families.

"In Gosport, where there are about sixty houses, some six hundred of the inhabitants reside, and among them may be classed some of the worst population of the town. The tenements . . . are exclusively occupied by Irish, of the very lowest description," he wrote. "They live huddled together in small close apartments, in which no regard is paid by them to cleanliness or to ventilation."[50]

Each room in each house was home to a family of Irish, so at least two hundred people lived in the eight buildings on Irish Row. These were not the days when people chose to live near the water, rather a time when the only place the poorest of the poor could afford were tenements shoddily built on the cheapest land around: hastily filled tidal marsh. The basements of the Irish apartments, though rarely completely dry, were home to small groceries or "groggeries," makeshift pubs. The marsh lapped at the rear of the lots, where the Irish often raised pigs and cows.

Trugien had been summoned to one of these apartments. In fact, the tenement fronted Water Street with the back lot abutting Page and Allen's dock. A resident, he'd been told, suffered from typical influenza symptoms: headache, fever, muscle pain, a debilitating backache. Trugien arrived to find not one but three people suffering from similar fevers.

He knew yellow fever, initially, could be tough to diagnose. The first blush of its symptoms could have indicated any number of fevers. Two of the victims recovered after a few days, showing no signs of problems after that, which gave Trugien no definitive answer. They'd each make the best of their luck and spend the rest of the summer nursing others sick with the fever. The third seemed to bounce back at first. He even returned to work at the Navy Yard and moved out of the sickly part of Gosport into a different part of Portsmouth.

Then his fever returned, which can happen to a small percentage of yellow fever victims. Sharp pain wrenched his stomach. His liver and kidneys slowed, and extra fluid from blood, urine, and waste backed up inside his body. He wretched—black-coffee-groundslike vomit. The expelled chunky fluid is only partly black, more a black and red porridge of blood that bursts from internal arteries and bubbles that look like tar. It smells like death.

The man died a few days after he relapsed. Schoolfield noted that he was a newcomer to the area, which gave the locals some comfort that it might not happen to them. But the jaundiced glaze over the victim's eyes, along with the yellow infusion of his skin, gave Trugien an undeniable answer: yellow fever.

Still, no one in town worried about the *Franklin*.

In early July, a machinist in his twenties, Robert Carter, took a steamer down the James River from Richmond looking for work. He had heard the shipyards had work for a tradesman like him. Carter rented a room on Water Street, about two hundred feet from the gates of the Navy Yard and two hundred feet from Page and Allen's Shipyard. He quickly landed work at Page and Allen's.

On Tuesday, July 3, Carter's first day on the job, the foreman sent him into the hold to help repair the *Franklin's* boilers. The next day, the shipyard closed for Independence Day, and Carter and some of his new workmates went to Old Point Comfort, the southern tip of the Virginia Peninsula where the Chesapeake Bay and Atlantic Ocean come together. It was an easy fifteen-mile boat ride from Gosport.[51]

Old Point, and its Hygeia hotel, attracted the rich and poor down through the years.[52] Edgar Allan Poe, President John Tyler, Andrew Jackson, and Henry Clay had all been there. Anne Phoebe Charlton Key, the sister of Frances Scott Key, stayed at the Hygeia during the summer of 1855.

Old Point had bowling, pistol shooting, and billiards. Carter and his friends, not having the funds to party inside the hotel with the well-off, would have joined hundreds of sunbathers at water's edge that day. They celebrated heavily, with plenty to drink.

When Carter didn't show up to work the next day, his coworkers figured he had overdone it. But he didn't turn up the day after that, either. On the morning of July 8, with Carter now running a fever, his head and back aching, his insides screaming, two Navy doctors and several other physicians came to examine him. In their foreign deployments, the military doctors had seen all kinds of fevers and symptoms.

They found a delirious Carter, his brain swollen from infection, his neck stiff, his head throbbing. One of the doctors reached down and pressed on his chest. Black vomit gurgled out of Carter. The doctors had no doubt; they were looking at a classic case of yellow fever. A few hours later, Carter died.[53]

The news flew around Portsmouth: A worker on the *Franklin* died of the fever. Even though it was Sunday, the Portsmouth Common Council called a meeting that afternoon. Angry and frightened residents packed the room.

The Navy doctors testified that they could with 100 percent confidence diagnose Carter's illness as yellow fever.

The captain dumped the bilge water on the pier, a resident called out.

He sent workers into the hold, others yelled.

The council proposed a resolution that the ship be sent back to quarantine. Captain Byram objected but only mildly because he knew the outcome. Council President Winchester Watts, after it was all said and done, wrote a letter to the *Franklin's* owners in New York detailing Byram's deceptions. In the end, the town sent the ship back to quarantine, and the shipping company replaced Byram.[54]

Schoolfield and others still had hope the fever could be contained. So far, there had been five cases, and three of the people had died. Then he learned of more.

When one of the three victims on Irish Row treated by Trugien fell sick, a friend from across the river in Hampton came to nurse her. Yellow fever seized that friend within a week, and she died five days later. John Cooke kept a small grocery in a dark, dank basement on Irish Row. Cooke died of the fever on July 10, and a woman who lived in the same house died the next day. Robert Allen and Ellen Conly, also residents of Irish Row, sickened and died a few days later. Still, fewer than ten victims were not enough to cause worry.

Schoolfield saw his first yellow fever case in Gosport on July 15. Jacob R. Race had arrived in Gosport two months earlier from New Jersey to join his friend William Mackey on a crew building a new ship at Page and Allen's. Schoolfield saw that Race displayed a textbook case of yellow fever, and he was dead five days later.

Mackey showed milder symptoms but was more alarmed at how the fever felled his friend so quickly. Mackey wanted to get far away and fast. He boarded a steamer up the Chesapeake Bay toward his home in New Jersey, but by the time he got to Baltimore illness forced him to halt his trip. He died before the end of the week.

Schoolfield wrestled with what he had seen. He looked for a reason to be hopeful that these dozen cases didn't portend the onset of a full-blown epidemic. It perplexed him that none of the people who had died after the machinist Carter had even been on the *Franklin*. If this ship was the source of the sickness, it didn't add up.

He found optimism in one commonality among the dead: "In every instance of death, the unfortunate individual was a newcomer," he wrote. "No native resident had yet died."[55]

That would not last much longer. The fever spread like a slow gas leak.

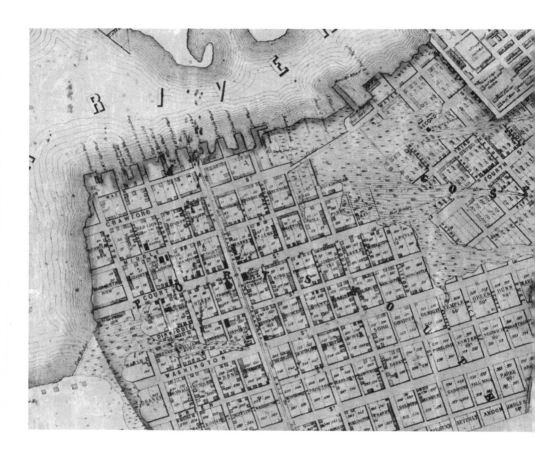

The central part of Portsmouth, Virginia, just across a footbridge
from the source of the outbreak, from James Keily's 1851 map.

CHAPTER FOUR

THE INFECTED DISTRICT

MOSQUITOES kill more people around the world every year than any other animal, and the second killer doesn't even come close. In most years, diseases transmitted by mosquitoes slay about three-quarters of a million people.[56] Yellow fever invaded the developed world beginning in the seventeenth century, dengue fever hit first in the nineteenth century, chikungunya in the twentieth century, followed by the emergence of Zika virus. The yellow fever mosquito, *Aedes aegypti*, carries all those deadly viruses.

Jeffrey R. Powell, a professor emeritus of ecology and evolutionary biology at Yale University, said the mosquito can likely ingest and transmit dozens of other viruses circulating in Africa right now.[57] It transmits disease almost invisibly. Powell calls the yellow fever mosquito "the most dangerous animal in the world."

As the residents of Norfolk and Portsmouth set out to stop the spread of the festering yellow fever outbreak, new cases hopping around town baffled them. The fever had, in fact, stowed away into the Virginia port on the *Franklin*, but not just in the form of stricken crew members and certainly not in the bad air released from the ship's belly.

Yellow fever originated deep in the jungles of Africa, in the equatorial rainforest that stretches like a wide belt across the fattest part of the continent. The region is so vast and remote that hundreds of years ago few if any people lived where the virus originated. The cycle begins when a female mosquito bites an infected monkey to siphon blood, which she needs to make her eggs strong. In ten to fifteen days, the virus strengthens enough inside her and when the mosquito draws blood from another monkey, it injects the monkey with it. Then other mosquitoes bite that monkey, and they get infected. The transmission nourishes itself and loops and loops and loops.

Mosquitoes adapt quickly, which is what makes them so fatal. They have an impressive determination to make sure their species survives and grows. Scientists aren't precisely sure when the yellow fever mosquito evolved to feed off people. Powell thinks mosquitoes most likely adapted to changes around them, when humans in West Africa began to build villages next to rainforests.[58] Swaths of West Africa experience droughts most years that last four to six months, and Powell figures a female mosquito looking for a place to deposit eggs during the dry months would take advantage of the drinking water stored in open containers around villages. That's when they would have, since they don't fly far, found a closer source for blood meals: people.

The eggs could have survived up to four months of drought, stuck to the side of containers, until the rains came. This change in how the species behaved—staying deep in the forest, others near villages—happened about four hundred to five hundred fifty years ago, Powell calculated. About that same time, in the 1600s, ships from European countries began docking in Western Africa to take the enslaved to the Americas. The ships would have resupplied their fresh water for the trip across the Atlantic Ocean from village supplies, in which the female mosquitoes had laid their eggs. When the mosquitoes hatched during the two- to four-month sail across the ocean, they would take wing to find a ship full of people to bite.

Aedes aegypti now had a hold in the New World. This species transformed into a legendary killing machine in densely settled villages and cities. Where their African cousins deposit eggs in the knots of trees or sunken spots in logs, the city mosquito *Aedes aegypti* hides her eggs in plain sight: clogged gutters, the saucer of a potted plant, a dried-out tire rut, a cistern, and certainly in the rain barrels that stored drinking water on ships' decks in 1855.

The indentation where the eggs are laid could be bone dry when the mosquito deposits them. A female mosquito lays her eggs at different levels above the water, in a clump of one hundred or so, where they stick to the side of the container. She'll lay others elsewhere—in a wheel rut, the divot made by a horse hoof, a puddle in the bottom of a boat. She'll lay several hundred in her short two to four weeks of life. The eggs remain viable even if it doesn't rain for as much as eight months. When it rains and the eggs get swamped, they float together like a little raft. Poof, in a few days, they hatch. In eight to ten days, they take wing.[59]

Aedes aegypti has evolved with fatal precision. Mosquitoes feed by day, especially during the first and last couple of hours of daylight, when people are most active. They can live outside or inside a home.

Eggs can survive and hatch even in brackish or salt water. On the *Franklin*, they would have bred in the salt water leaked into the ship's hull on its way from Saint Thomas to Portsmouth. With crew members sick with yellow fever before leaving the West Indies, healthy mosquitoes that hatched on the way up the Atlantic Coast feasted on the men infected with the virus.

The transmission cycle would've been in full bloom when they docked. By the nineteenth century, the yellow fever mosquito had become native to coastal Virginia. Infected people who left the ship passed the virus along to the local mosquitoes that bit them. Schoolfield was half right in his optimistic note that only nonnative people had sickened early on because if a person had ever contracted yellow fever and lived, they would be immune for the rest of their lives. The nonnative immigrants would not likely have been exposed to yellow fever in Ireland, so they were susceptible.

What Schoolfield didn't understand is that few "native" Virginians had gotten and survived yellow fever. The last serious epidemic to hit Norfolk and Portsmouth was in 1826, three decades earlier. The Irish newcomers and the unexposed locals combined to create two cities of twenty-six thousand people who had almost no immunity. They were fresh meat.

With few immune residents, there were no dead ends, no roadblocks to slow the virus. Almost every person a mosquito bit became a mobile reservoir of the virus, carrying it to a different cluster of *Aedes aegypti* in a new part of town.

The ship had lit a match. The cities were like a prairie of dry grass.

ON THE THIRD week of July, cases of yellow fever sprouted in the middle of Portsmouth. It were as if the virus bored a tunnel from the Gosport waterfront and across the marsh, then popped out of a hole several blocks away.

Everyone expected if the fever spread, it logically would move from house to house, then block to block. Yet here it was, at the city farmer's market next to High Street smack-dab in the middle of town. Five of the first six people to catch the fever there died. At the same time, the people of Portsmouth lost another of the protections they had been counting on; more than newcomers were dying. The fever started to fell locals, too.

Frederick Godwin was not new to the area, nor did he live in a cramped apartment. He lived with his father in Gosport. The Godwin house stood off by itself, on a high, dry foundation with plenty of fresh breezes passing through the windows. Yellow fever attacked Godwin on July 19, as far as doctors could tell, but it must've been savaging him internally before that. He quickly became delirious and dropped into a coma. Three days later, he died. Within days, Godwin's sister, brother-in-law, then four other members of the Godwin family caught yellow fever and died.[60]

All of them were Virginia natives and had lived in town for many years. None had been on board the *Franklin.*

Despite the Market Street outbreak, Portsmouth residents swung into high gear to try again to cordon off the spread into what they called the "infected district." They stationed police officers at the footbridge to Gosport. The police stood guard twenty-four hours a day. Frightened residents even tore down part of the bridge. They were only concerned about people moving in one direction, from Gosport to Portsmouth. Doctors like Schoolfield and Trugien, nurses, and ministers visiting sick members of their flocks still forayed into the sick part of town. Residents, though, didn't have to be convinced to stay away from the shipyards and Irish tenements.

Quarantining or isolating the sick goes back at least nine hundred years, to a bubonic plague in Venice, Italy, in 1127, and probably back to the days of leprosy. Finding some way to separate the sick from the well has been attempted in nearly every disease outbreak in human history.[61] In 1636, during the bubonic plague in London that killed more than ten thousand people, England mandated that households with sick people be shuttered or have the sick carted to pest houses until they recovered or died. Towns appointed "searchers" to look for houses where someone had succumbed to the plague. When they found a victim, a constable would padlock the house shut, even if people were still alive inside. Those running the country, city, or town under siege considered the tactics necessary for everyone's protection. Those being quarantined felt like they were punished for being sick.[62] After just three weeks, it had already come to this in Portsmouth.

On July 20, the Portsmouth Common Council acted. They appointed a Sanitary Committee consisting of three men and gave them the power to take whatever measures necessary to slow or stop the "impending calamity." They appointed Schoolfield as chairman, an obvious choice since he'd already been doing the job. In addition to cordoning off Gosport, the committee dispatched people to go house by house through the town to inspect every street and every lot and remove sources of filth. To absorb the odors in the bad air they believed to be spreading yellow fever, they dumped five hundred barrels of lime sulfate in yards and on the streets.[63]

The Sanitary Committee decided that direct information might reduce the residents' fears. They requested that each of the eight doctors in town document their cases and deaths at sunset every day so the committee could provide daily reports on "the state of the prevailing epidemic."

The committee released its first report on July 24:

"FROM THE RETURNS of three physicians, there were under treatment at sunset on the 23rd, eighteen cases. Up to the present time there have been eight deaths only. The disease is principally confined to Gosport, there being only a few cases in other parts of town, and they originated in Gosport.

J.N. SCHOOLFIELD, Chairman."[64]

Until the morning of July 29, Portsmouth residents figured they had corralled the outbreak. It had been a full month since Trugien diagnosed the first cases of yellow fever on Irish Row, a couple hundred feet from where the *Franklin* had docked for repairs. The Sanitary Committee report from the evening before, its fifth report so far, revealed ten new cases of the fever in Gosport and four deaths. People didn't know that most doctors in Portsmouth were so swamped with yellow fever patients that they hadn't had time to report to the committee. Trugien routinely moved around town treating people from sunrise until 9 p.m.

People aren't good at sizing up danger, especially evaluating a threat in real time. When a whole town, in its collective fear and wishful thinking, assesses peril, information becomes distorted like light refracting through a prism. Portsmouth's residents had convinced themselves that the illness was an Irish problem that could be herded back into that part of town or at least somewhere that barely inconvenienced the rest of them. But by the morning of July 29 in Portsmouth, the signs of a festering yellow fever outbreak had become clear as daybreak.

That Sunday just after sunrise, a group of Irish from Gosport were hanging around in the enclosed courtyard of the Academy. That was right downtown, catacorner from the Presbyterian Church, two blocks from the courthouse and just steps from High Street, the backbone of the town's commerce. It had been a sweltering night, the thermometer barely dipping even after sunset, and people slept with their windows open to get any air they could. Shortly after dawn, it hit eighty degrees.[65] The sultry air, it seemed, had flushed everyone out onto their porches or into the streets. Word spread quickly about the Irish loitering downtown. This couldn't stand. Reverend James Chisholm, minister of Saint John's Episcopal, described what happened next: "Soon a gathering of citizens from various quarters takes place, and the excitement occasioned by the apprehension that the Academy is about to become a rendezvous for members from the seat of infection becomes so great that the Irish all leave the spot. However, these poor creatures received every humane attention, and good food and clean clothing came to them in abundance from various families from this and neighboring streets." Chisholm didn't have any food or clothes to contribute, he wrote to his wife, so he donated a dollar, worth about thirty-five dollars today.

At the Sanitary Committee's urging, the townspeople had spent the past forty-eight hours nailing together a twenty-foot-by-forty-foot "pest house" over by a cemetery to haul the sick and dying Irish out of the tenements for nursing care; not to mention, a place where they'd be safely away from everyone else. Even healthy residents of Irish Row would have to leave so their apartments could be thoroughly "whitewashed" with calcified lime. For good measure, town stewards would wipe the surfaces with thieves vinegar, a concoction of wine, herbs, garlic, and spices that surely would keep most (other) bad smells away.

It was the same situation on Water Street in Gosport. A horde of self-appointed patrollers figured the only way to hem in the surging outbreak was to remove the sick. The terrified Irish families wouldn't budge. Chisholm and others were furious. The way Chisholm saw it, first, that same morning they'd clustered over at the Academy and had to be run off. Now, they spurned the town's generosity in building a pest house for them to recover in. Chisholm's disgust sniveled from his pen when he wrote to his wife later that evening: "The wretched and squalid patients in Irish Row positively refused to abandon their pestilential abodes. These, in number between three hundred and four hundred, reeking in nameless abomination and filth and stench, and exhibiting in their conduct towards one another a hard-heartedness of which we would not have dared to believe human nature capable under such circumstances, reveling and fighting and quarrelling amongst the dying and over the dead, they refuse to stir."[66]

Portsmouth residents had no idea they couldn't halt the spread of the fever by fencing in the people who had it or that when they relocated the sick they were transplanting virus hot spots to other parts of town. The next day, they were back at the Gosport waterfront across from Page and Allen's wharf to evict the Irish families. In this part of town, the greatest commercial vulnerability lay a few hundred feet down Water Street: the massive Gosport Navy Yard, a critical asset for the whole country with the nation's first dry dock. Whatever means were needed, it would be best for Portsmouth, Norfolk across the river, and truly, the entire country if the town could repel the fever from the Navy Yard. The convening horde that morning included townspeople, doctors, ministers, servants, and the enslaved. Since they needed someone the Irish would listen to, they sent for Reverend Francis Devlin, priest at Saint Paul's Roman Catholic Church. Though he had Mass in another hour, he sensed the rising tension and hurried down Water Street, across the marsh on the causeway.

Looking over the gathered crowd, feeling the anxiousness and impatience, the priest feared for the young families. He saw no option, at least none the increasingly hostile masses would tolerate, other than for the Irish families to leave. With the backing of the doctors, he convinced the tenement residents to take the irrefusable offer. Devlin and the doctors helped the people crawl up onto wooden carts for a hot, jostling ride over bumpy streets to the pest house. Everyone sensed it was the moment when things turned. Even Chisholm could see the grimness of the scene: "A most melancholy spectacle is the removal, under the noon-day heat of an almost tropical sun. Nine carts were filled with sufferers, in some cases two to a cart, lying prostrate, in others, three or four sitting. Their agonized faces and their piteous groans awakened mingled horrors and compassion."

Several of the Irish families had not waited for the townsfolk to return that day. They'd seen before how things would play out. With the threat that Irish Row would be boarded up, they gathered their belongings, caught the ferry, and moved in with friends or relatives across the river. Many of them flopped onto apartment floors of an Irish enclave called Barry's Row, down by the water in Norfolk.

The removal of the sick, and the eviction of the others, had unintended consequences. It sent the fear of God and the fever shivering through everyone in town. The makeshift hospital, or pest house, had been erected at the far edge of the main part of Portsmouth by Portlock Cemetery. The carts loaded with suffering, moaning people meandered their way through town for all to see. One particular wagon drew the eyes of everyone out on the streets that day. Covered in white cloth to shield the sun, with a mattress on its bed, it carried just a mother and daughter in the back. The husband and father had died hours earlier. Everyone on the crowded sidewalks stopped and stared. No one spoke. They stood in silence even after it passed. Schoolfield called that day, August 1, "the blackest day on which the sun ever shone in the history of Portsmouth."[67]

"What had been feared and hoped against had now become a

reality," he wrote, "and each of us felt that he was living and moving in the midst of a pestilence."

No longer could anyone deny the existence of the fever, nor downplay its effect on victims. And it certainly wasn't just an Irish problem.

Portsmouth residents weren't yet aware of what was happening around the country: Much like they'd tried to wall off Gosport, the rest of the East Coast cities were staking the equivalent of a massive seine net in the waters around Portsmouth and Norfolk. Though many of the lessons learned from the Philadelphia epidemics were not the right ones, the people in port cities saw what they saw when yellow fever broke out. And what they saw time and again, for the past century, was that it started on ships. New York went first in throwing up a quarantine to ban ships from Norfolk and Portsmouth. The *New York Times* published the news under the simple headline "Quarantine" on July 29:

> "IN VIEW OF the existence of cholera and yellow fever at the ports of Norfolk and Portsmouth, Va., Isaac O. Barker, acting mayor in the absence of Mayor Wood, has issued the following proclamation: Whereas from reliable information received from the ports of Norfolk and Portsmouth, in Virginia, this department is advised that the yellow fever now prevails in both of these parts. Be it therefore known to all men that by virtue of the power vested, and by and with the advice and consent of the Board of Commissioners of Health of this port, I, Isaac O. Barker, Acting Mayor of the City of New York, do issue this proclamation, declaring said ports of Norfolk and Portsmouth, in the State of Virginia, as infected places and all vessels arriving from said places to be subjected to Quarantine."

The new quarantine instantly sidelined the steamer *Roanoke* in the New York harbor. After that, quarantines against Norfolk and Portsmouth flew up: Baltimore, which had daily steamer service down the Chesapeake Bay to Norfolk; Petersburg, Virginia; and nearby Hampton and Suffolk. Even neighboring Isle of Wight County banned people from the twin cities. The county had become a haven for people who lacked the money to travel by steamer or rail. Fleeing families would lug whatever possessions they could load on a cart and build makeshift camps in the woods and fields. Fistfights broke out among Isle of Wight locals and the refugees, with the locals scared that those fleeing had brought the fever with them.

At Old Point Comfort, a sliver of land that pokes out into the Chesapeake Bay just a few miles from Norfolk, the Army commandant in charge stationed sentries with bayonets on the piers to repel boats coming from Norfolk or Portsmouth. Philadelphia had suffered more yellow fever outbreaks than any other American city over the years. Despite the opinion of the Revolutionary-era hero Doctor Benjamin Rush that the cause of the epidemics was local, the city had seen too many occasions when the fever erupted a few weeks after a foreign ship docked. The papers reported on August 6:

"PHILADELPHIA—The Board of Health has passed a resolution that, until otherwise ordered, all vessels coming to this port, including steamers from Norfolk and Portsmouth, Va., shall stop at the Lazaretto station, for the purpose of receiving a visit from the physician of that place before coming up to the city."

On July 30, the mayor of Baltimore and the city's health commissioners visited Norfolk and Portsmouth to see for themselves. Twenty cases and four deaths had been reported overnight. Unlike other cities, Baltimore would not rely on reports from the press that lagged by days or rumors from frightened residents. Authorities ordered that "skillful physicians be placed on both the Norfolk boats, to prevent any sick persons being brought on board, and with the power to detain the boats or passengers at Quarantine if necessary."

Richmond's actions stung the most. Richmond and Norfolk were each other's closest trading partners, with steamers carrying passengers and goods back and forth daily, a mail boat that also swapped the days' newspapers from each city, and a telegraph wire that offered instant communications before its operator quit. The *Richmond Dispatch* saw what was coming and pleaded for logic: "Richmond bears the same relation to Norfolk that Columbia, in South Carolina, does to Charleston. The disease prevails annually in Charleston, but though there is constant and large communication between Charleston and Columbia, the inhabitants of the latter place never suffer from it. It is the opinion of the majority of the medical profession that the yellow fever never prevails except in malarious districts. If this be so there is no cause for alarm in Richmond."[68]

Regardless, the Richmond Council met August 1 at 4 p.m., just two days after New York erected a quarantine. It acted fast. Richmond didn't have a designated quarantine area but delineated one on the James River near Hancock's Island. Just as quickly, the council created the position of superintendent of quarantine and voted a man into that role. Then the councilmen got down to the reason they convened and unanimously adopted a resolution to barricade the cities downriver:

"IMPORTANT NOTICE to Vessels—Resolved, that until otherwise ordered by the Council of the city of Richmond, all sail and steam vessels of whatever class, coming from or touching at either of the ports of Norfolk, Portsmouth or Gosport, shall be subjected to quarantine limits for the port of the city of Richmond."[69]

With that, it would still be possible to leave Norfolk and Portsmouth, but it would require more maneuvering—and more uncertainty. Even if a boat continued to run its route, would its destination permit it to dock? Would the passengers be allowed to disembark? Or would it be rebuffed and sent back home? The residents of the twin cities weren't trapped yet, but their options for leaving worsened with each trip of the steamers. Their best hope, it seemed to many, was to get out before other East Coast cities had the chance to stop them.

Before the sun had fully risen that Friday morning, August 3, it seemed like every man, woman, and child in Portsmouth was on the move[70]—horses loaded with bags, porters laden with trunks, wheelbarrows, carts, suitcases, boxes, entire families scurrying together in amoebalike blobs, parents hauling small children in their arms or walking-almost-running as they nearly dragged them by their hands toward the wharf. Where every side road or alley intersected with High Street, families appeared almost as apparitions through the gray fumes of smoking tar barrels and converged into the stream of panicked people. Cart wheels rattled over cobblestones, dogs barked, neighbors hollered as they bustled, creating a swirling cacophony of fright.

Winchester Watts, president of Portsmouth's Town Council, wrote to his brother, who had already fled town with his family: "I have never before witnessed such a scene in the way of panic as was exhibited this morning at the railroad yard wharf nearly an hour before departure of the boat. The whole wharf was strewn with trunks, carpet bags and crowded with a dense mass of human beings of all ages and conditions." So many people huddled on the wharf that Watts feared the boat couldn't hold them all or that they'd be crushed when the mass of humans surged toward the gate. Before the crew even had the steamer lashed to the pier, those at the front of the crowd pushed and squeezed to hop on board.

Watts had already decided to stay behind, out of a sense of duty, but told his brother not to return. "Most of the stores are closed and the market but slimly attended. Our town already begins to wear a most gloomy and somber aspect. I fear that if this state of things should continue, our town will be almost de-populated."[71]

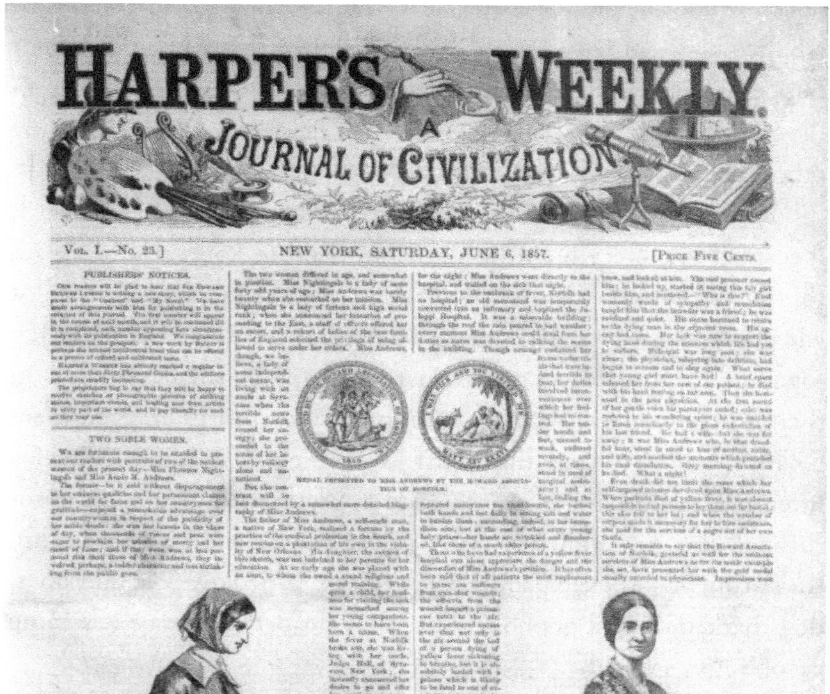

HARPER'S WEEKLY.
A JOURNAL OF CIVILIZATION.

VOL. I.—No. 23.] NEW YORK, SATURDAY, JUNE 6, 1857. [PRICE FIVE CENTS.

PUBLISHERS' NOTICES.

TWO NOBLE WOMEN.

MEDAL PRESENTED TO MISS ANDREWS BY THE HOWARD ASSOCIATION OF NORFOLK.

FLORENCE NIGHTINGALE.

ANNIE M. ANDREWS.—[FROM AN AMBROTYPE BY BRADY.]

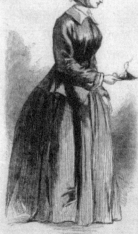

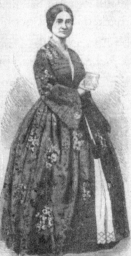

Annie Andrews, lower right, as shown on the front page of *Harper's Weekly Journal of Civilization.*

CHAPTER FIVE
LEAPING THE RIVER

I N July, a young woman in Syracuse, New York, named Annie M. Andrews began reading in "the mail from the South" news about a yellow fever outbreak. Each time the mail arrived, the news worsened. She became set on traveling to the sick cities to help.[72]

Her friends begged her not to go. A woman not even twenty-five, traveling by herself? Anything could happen. Where would she stay? Was it safe? Would she be able to get food to cook? She wasn't sure, but she penned a letter to Norfolk's new mayor, Hunter Woodis, volunteering her services. Cleverly, Woodis did not accept her offer. Instead he wrote back with a detailed description of the devastation he was already seeing and how the fever afflicted the city more and more each day. He cautioned her that if she came, he could make no promises about her housing or food. He'd do his best, but the grocers and banks already talked of shutting.[73]

"He shrank from the responsibility of advising me to risk my life there," Andrews concluded, "and he also shrank from rejecting my service to those so sorely in need of help."

Andrews was the daughter of a New Orleans businessman. Having grown up in New Orleans meant she could have been bitten by a mosquito carrying yellow fever, survived, and become immune.

Whatever the case, she did not wait for additional instructions or approval from Woodis. She had been staying with her uncle in Syracuse, where in addition to her personal correspondences with Southern friends she would have read of the burgeoning epidemic in the *New York Times* and the Syracuse papers. She headed south.

Andrews took a train to Baltimore, where she transferred to the steamer *Georgia*, one of the ships of the Baltimore Steam Packet Company, nicknamed the Old Bay Line.[74] She quickly overheard talk suggesting she was sailing into the teeth of a calamity more severe than she thought. "What's the news?" she heard one passenger ask another from the stricken cities. The matter-of-fact litany of woe shocked Andrews: "We put away so and so last night," or "Mrs. So and so has fallen victim." [75]

On the trip south, Andrews met three Catholic volunteers from Emmitsburg, Maryland, a community known as the Sisters of Charity. The Emmitsburg sisterhood would become the mother tree of similar ones from Canada and New York all the way to Bermuda. Andrews, Sister Christine, Sister Susannah, and Sister Mary would work hand-in-hand throughout the summer, becoming the first of many nurses and doctors to volunteer in Norfolk and Portsmouth. Andrews had arrived so early in the crisis, on the same boat as the Sisters, that most in town assumed she also was Catholic.

Though the work was grim, they wanted to get started right away. As soon as they dragged their bags off the *Georgia*, they found a hack and a horse-drawn taxi and went in search of Mayor Woodis. It didn't take long. "He was pointed out to us by the hackman, who beckoned to him and drove up," Andrews remembered. Woodis quickly impressed her, with an unassuming but direct manner, a cordial handshake, and what she thought was a "noble face."[76]

Unlike in Portsmouth, no public announcement had been made of the first cases of yellow fever in Norfolk. By the third week of July, the chatter around town strongly suggested it. On July 30, as Chisholm and others were rounding up the Irish in Gosport, a

Norfolk correspondent for the *Richmond Dispatch* broke the news about what everyone in town already feared.

"The yellow fever, as might have been expected, made its appearance in our city, notwithstanding every precaution was taken to prevent the spread of the disease from Gosport," he wrote. "I understand that the disease was brought here by a woman who escaped from the infected district at Gosport."

In the same report, the correspondent, who filed his stories under the pen name MARINER, wrote about the Sisters of Charity's arrival. "Should death thin their ranks, or the disease spread very rapidly, they will be reinforced from Emmitsburg, Maryland."[77]

Norfolk, being the larger of the two, usually had more resources than its sister city across the river, and early in the outbreak this showed. Norfolk had already converted the buildings at an old horse racing track called Julappi into a makeshift hospital. Doctors at the hospital, at the edge of the Elizabeth River, figured the fresh breeze would improve sufferers' health. Mayor Woodis arranged for a carriage and took Andrews out to what they now called Julappi Hospital.[78]

After Andrews served at Julappi a few days, Woodis and Doctor George Upshur sent for her to help the fever-afflicted in town. Upshur had treated the first cases in Norfolk in Barry's Row, the Irish tenements down in swampy land by the river. Few knew it other than Upshur and the mayor, but people in Norfolk had begun falling ill with suspicious symptoms as early as July 16.

The Irish Row tenements over in Gosport were most assuredly poorly built, not maintained by the landlord, and unkempt. Barry's Row was not to be outdone. Its residents had been charged exorbitant rent, so they jammed as many families into each unit as possible. The ground on which the buildings sat had been tidal marsh a decade earlier, and they now sat on "made land." But water stubbornly returns to where it's meant to be. During abnormally high tides, or after heavy rains ran off into the streets and the tide came in, water oozed up through the planks in first-floor units at Barry's Row.

On that day, the carriage brought Andrews to Barry's Row, where Woodis and Upshur met her. Norfolk, too, had embraced the optimistic idea that the virus lived within an infected district and that lives could be saved by keeping people out of that part of town. It made a degree of sense: In earlier epidemics, the virus had not spread north of Main Street. Many people, including Upshur, relocated out of downtown early in the outbreak to live with friends or relatives north of the imagined edge of the infected district. What they didn't understand is that in previous years, such as the last big epidemic in 1826, the fever hadn't spread beyond Main Street simply because not many people lived there yet.

Andrews knew Woodis had been removing the sick from Barry's Row, not in a forceful way like across the river but to get them help. She had cared for them when they arrived at Julappi. She now saw how Woodis intended to halt the burgeoning outbreak: hammering boards together to wall off Barry's Row.

While Andrews watched, a bunch of locals came by to protest the barrier. How could Woodis cut off their path to other parts of town?

"It shall not go up!" they told him.

Woodis was calm, assertive, and fearless, Andrews thought.

"It shall go up," Woodis told them, "and what's more, it shall remain up. I'll watch here night by night."

And that was the end of it. Upshur, known for his quick wit, nicknamed the fence "The Woodis Board of Health."[79]

Jokes aside, Woodis and his new Know Nothings-dominated City Council could not agree on how to appoint watchmen to stand guard at the wooden barricades. Some of the guards had been a little too enthusiastic for the opportunity to block the path of the Irish residents. One man, an acquaintance of the *Dispatch* correspondent MARINER, had been a watchman one night and came out the next night without being asked. He got so aggressive in stopping passersby that the appointed watchmen had him arrested and thrown in jail for the night. Instead of consulting with the council, Woodis decided he would hand-select the sentries.

Though the *Dispatch* was printing bulletins from Norfolk correspondents, none of the local papers had yet reported on the yellow fever outbreak. MARINER, a correspondent, hit upon the reason in a late July post:

"Business of every description is dull; and now that the yellow fever has broken out on this side, and it is likely to become an epidemic, trade, it is feared, will become completely stagnant. Various reports, mostly exaggerated, are flying around about it."

On July 30, Upshur made public that he had been treating sick people in Barry's Row and that his most recent case had left no doubt that they were stricken with yellow fever. As Upshur knew it would, divulging the news made him the bad guy to just about everyone. The public was already anxious, terrified of the unknown and what might happen. Some blamed the doctor for not coming out with the news sooner so they could have acted swiftly to limit the spread by removing victims beyond the city limits and ramping up disinfecting the streets and alleys.

Many others wished Upshur had kept his mouth shut. The news would stifle business even more than the rumors, they thought. Wait until the northern newspapers latched onto this. They called Upshur an alarmist and bitterly dubbed the illness the "Upshur Fever." Whichever the case, Upshur's pronouncement caused a flurry of worry among Norfolk residents. Trugien had treated the first cases in Gosport on June 30. Now, just thirty-one days later, the fever had leapt the Elizabeth River, the only real barrier between the two cities.

It was August 1 when Reverend George Armstrong sat at a desk in his house, dipped his pen in ink, and began jotting notes in his journal about the outbreak. His words show he was anxious about what might unfold. Yet, much like when a hurricane or blizzard brews in the distance, he was a bit excited about the mystery and the chance to really show his flock his dedication. Like many in Norfolk, Armstrong was a newcomer.

He was born in Mendham, New Jersey, about forty miles west of New York City. His father was a Presbyterian minister. His mother, Polly, raised him and his nine brothers and sisters. George was fascinated by how the world around him worked, attracted to the sciences, and attended Princeton College, graduating at age nineteen. Afterward, he moved to Richmond to live with his brother, who was also a minister. His brother persuaded him to pursue the ministry in addition to scientific studies. Armstrong attended seminary and became ordained in 1837. He moved to the quiet Shenandoah Valley town of Lexington, Virginia.[80]

There, he preached at a small church and taught at Washington College, now Washington and Lee University, where he became a professor of chemistry and mechanics. By 1851, one of the largest Presbyterian churches in the South, First Presbyterian in Norfolk, needed a minister and they summoned Armstrong. The church demanded all his time and attention, and he no longer could teach. But he kept up with scientific theory by corresponding with former colleagues and professors and extensive newspaper and book reading. His scientific background and analytical mind made him an astute observer of the simmering outbreak. If things went badly, he figured there would be a need for objective eyewitness accounts.

Armstrong was friends with Upshur, who was a deacon at First Presbyterian. Armstrong had no doubt that Upshur's diagnoses of the first cases had put him in an unenviable spot and that Upshur had acted responsibly reporting them when he did. Still, Armstrong noted that the Upshur announcement "caused no little excitement among our people, in fact, many families are already leaving our city." Armstrong attributed the flight to the fear of the unknown since three decades had passed since the last serious epidemic in Norfolk. In cities where the fever appears almost annually, he said, it doesn't cause as much excitement.

"For those who are disposed to take the most cheerful view, it is said this fever appears to be of a very mild and manageable type,"

he wrote. The city's Board of Health had reported that morning that there had been "only" seventeen cases in fourteen days, with three of them resulting in death.[81]

Like many, Armstrong had been told that the major outbreaks of 1822 and 1826 had plagued only the blocks down by the water, now known as the infected district. "In those years, persons living in that district had just to remove to the north of Main Street, and they were as safe from the fever as they would have been a thousand miles off," Armstrong wrote in his journal.[82]

He was optimistic for other more logical reasons. In the past ten years, Norfolk had paved nearly all its streets. This would have been done with a new method developed by a Scottish engineer named John Loudon McAdam: a foundation of crushed rock, packed after each layer by a cast-iron roller, then topped with either finely crushed stone or sand. The roads were ten to eighteen inches deep and firm enough to withstand horse hooves and wagon wheels even after a rain.[83]

During the citywide paving, even though Norfolk seemed flat, they graded the streets into a subtle slope. So now horse manure, discarded food, fish guts from the market, and whatever else eventually washed down into the river.

"Norfolk is now one of the most thoroughly paved cities in the Union," Armstrong wrote. "The streets have been so carefully graded that water runs off almost as soon as it does in Richmond, with all its hills. A careful comparison of our bills of mortality with those of other cities will show that for the last ten years, Norfolk has been one of the healthiest cities on the Atlantic seaboard."

People were going around town looking for filth and anything else unsanitary. Armstrong thought now that everyone knew yellow fever had a foothold in the city, people were more "sharp-sighted than usual" and noticed street detritus they would normally have looked past.[84]

He tended to think his way around issues. It was as if he would have to debate himself in writing, taking great pains to lay out the strongest argument of each side, go back and forth a couple of times, then land at a decision. He wanted to remain hopeful, but he also saw a lot of potential danger in what lay before the city.

Rumors flew that more than one type of yellow fever existed, and the fact that a high percentage of the first people to catch the fever in Portsmouth and Norfolk died did not bode well. "It is said," Armstrong wrote, "the fever now existing in our midst is not the ordinary yellow fever, but the African fever that is a traveling epidemic . . . and has been gradually making its way north along the Atlantic coast."

Armstrong was right, in a way. Plotted on a map, major outbreaks did appear to be working their way up the coast from Rio de Janeiro in 1849 and 1850, to New Orleans in 1853, on to Savannah, Georgia, the following year, and now Norfolk and Portsmouth.

The epidemic in Rio erupted after the British government began pressuring Brazil to end the slave trade. The threat prompted ships to bolt to the Brazilian coast full of captives from Africa to supply the exploding demand for labor in the country's coffee and sugar farms. Even as the death rate hit eighty and then ninety people a day, the government tried to protect trade and kept the port open. Doctors suggested shooting artillery into the sky and lighting bonfires in the streets to cleanse the sick air. In the end, yellow fever slayed four thousand one hundred sixty people in the city of one hundred sixty-six thousand.[85]

In New Orleans, yellow fever broke out nearly every year. In 1847, it killed two thousand residents, but for the next five years it killed only a couple hundred each summer. The city had been draining and filling swamps to remove sources of bad air, and confidence had grown that major outbreaks were a thing of the past. The *New Orleans Medical and Surgical Journal* wrote in 1852 that the day would soon come when "the existence of that disease will be known only in the recollection of older inhabitants." The following year, in 1853, another fever epidemic erupted. The papers did not report its existence until two months after the first cases, after one thousand people had died. All told that year, yellow fever killed 7,849 people.

In Savannah, Georgia, the 1854 epidemic took one thousand forty lives after a ship from Havana arrived. The outbreak was marked by a hurricane that struck in early September, swamping the city and setting off a mosquito bloom. The second noteworthy element of the Savannah eruption was its toll on those treating the victims: Ten doctors and ten medical students died.

In Norfolk, the human urge to gather the family, stock up on supplies, and hunker down faced off with a powerful counter-urge to throw what they needed into duffels or trunks and run for their lives. When the unfolding calamity was yellow fever, fleeing until the first frost was the only surefire preventative.

If the population wasn't terrified enough, the *Richmond Dispatch* published a lengthy piece in late July under the heading "Epidemics" about previous scourges going back to the Middle Ages. The paper recounted Black Death, the plague that hopscotched around medieval Europe and killed between seventy-five million and two hundred million people. In 1665, the plague struck London, taking more than sixty-five thousand lives, perhaps as many as one hundred thousand— one out of every five Londoners. The *Dispatch* put a fine point on the relevance, reminding readers of the "terrific power of certain unknown agents of mortality, which there is reason to fear still exist."

As Armstrong went around town visiting parishioners, he saw that each day, on each block, another house or two would be empty. He saw families stricken with fear hauling their children and whatever else they thought they'd need for a couple of months on the way to the wharves. He didn't like it, but he understood.

If he thought the lethal strain of yellow fever that devastated New Orleans two years ago and Savannah last year had taken root in Norfolk and Portsmouth, he'd pray that every single resident got as far away as they could.

"With two long, hot months which must intervene between this and frost, it must make terrible havoc," Armstrong thought. "In the prospect of such a possibility, I can only say 'God help us, for the help of man is vain.'"

Armstrong and his wife, Mehetable, had discussed the risks. They had three daughters: Twelve-year-old Mary, ten-year-old Cornelia, and eight-year-old Grace. Mehetable's sister and nephew also lived with them.

Armstrong thought that times like these were what called someone to become a leader. If the heavens did unfurl a cataclysmic, citywide epidemic, his parishioners would face one of the most daunting and terrifying events of their lives. If he left them to their own fates now, he wouldn't be much of a pastor.

"No mere danger to themselves personally should enter into the decision," Armstrong wrote on that August 1. "My own convictions of duty were never plainer than they are at this time."

He and his family would stay in town "come what may."

CHAPTER SIX

PHILADELPHIA: THE DAMAGE DONE

ON the morning of August 19, 1793, three doctors stood at the bedside of a patient who lay struggling to breathe in her home near the Philadelphia wharves. Peter LeMaigre had threaded himself into the fabric of the city after thirty years as an importer and international merchant. His plea for medical help for his wife, Catherine, had summoned a crack team: Doctor John Foulke, a fellow of the prominent College of Physicians and a physician at Pennsylvania Hospital; Doctor Hugh Hodge, a surgeon in the Revolutionary War; and Doctor Benjamin Rush, a wunderkind who graduated from the College of New Jersey (later Princeton University) at age fourteen and went on to earn a medical degree at the University of Edinburgh in Scotland, the world's best for medical training.

At age forty-seven, Rush was well-known throughout the country: By the time he was twenty-three, he had established a medical practice and taught chemistry at the College of Philadelphia. Politically, Thomas Paine consulted Rush on Paine's pro-independence writings, Rush was a signatory on the Declaration of Independence, and Rush was adamantly in favor of abolishing slavery. During the Revolutionary War, he earned credibility with the troops when he embedded with the Pennsylvania Militia to tend to battle wounds and sickness.[86]

Now, on this August morning in 1793, Rush was about to diagnose a case that would make him the most famous doctor in America for the next half century.

Rush had already gained fame, or infamy, for his controversial medical theories. Among other things, he was convinced that sickness was fairly simple: The single root of all human illness was fever. And the cause of all fever was foul air. That August 19 morning, he was already stirred up about the stinking city. On his way to the LeMaigre house, he had skirted the High Street market where the remnants of yesterday's sales lay in the street. The stench smacked his senses: sheep heads, cattle entrails, animal manure, decaying vegetables, all left to rot or be picked at by vultures, gulls, and stray dogs. If the streets were cleaned up, Rush thought, and the smell of decay gone, health problems like the flu, whooping cough, yellow fever, and even cancer would vanish.[87] In fact, a few years earlier, he had announced that he'd discovered a new medical fundamental: Regardless of the various disease names, all sicknesses in the world originated from just one fever—the result of convulsive blood vessels. The only thing that could calm the hyperactive blood vessels was frequent bleeding and purging.[88]

The LeMaigre house itself perched on a street that hardly seemed habitable. Water Street, a street in name only, was more like an afterthought of a swampy alley. "The narrowest, yet one of the most populous streets in the city. The street is only thirty feet wide, and but a little above the surface of the tide: the houses are high, and the greater part of them have no yards. It is much confined, ill-aired, and, in every respect, is a disagreeable street."

Among them, the three doctors had seen a lot of sickness, and they all could see that it was too late for Catherine LeMaigre. She lay in bed, her chest heaving up and down with shallow breaths. She was gagging up black vomit. Huddled together, the doctors recounted that since early August each of them had treated an unusual number of people with similar symptoms: severe fever, nausea, nervous pulses, black vomit—and often, tinted yellow skin.

Rush had lost a patient the day before, the twenty-five-year-old wife of a good friend. She had died of a violent fever. And those weren't the first signs, as Rush put it, "that all was not right with our city." Two weeks earlier, another doctor had called Rush for a consultation on a young girl who was feverish and vomiting. Rush noticed a yellowish tint to her skin. That same week, he'd been called to see a printer friend's wife, with bloodshot eyes, a headache, and nausea. Rush was among the medical profession's loudest advocates for bloodletting, a practice he suggested both to maintain good health as well as to cure acute diseases. As proof of his conviction, he routinely lanced and drained blood from himself. His detractors sniggered that his chronic cough made him a shining example of why not to bloodlet. But it was Rush's go-to treatment. He bled the printer's wife twice and gave her a dose of calomel, mercury chloride. She somehow survived.

The more they talked, the doctors realized their cases had all arisen from houses in the Water Street area. As they pondered, they would have looked out windows at the wharves. Doctor Foulke spoke up.

This stale, noxious smell in the air had an obvious origin, Foulke said. The sloop *Amelia* had arrived in late July from Saint-Domingue, crowded with refugees. A load of coffee had rotted along the way, and the crew had dumped the coffee beans onto a wharf. There, it had continued to decompose "to the great annoyance of the whole neighborhood." It was as if Rush had been slapped in the face. His nose for noxiousness smelled a discovery.

All Rush's patients and others he had heard about had lived within a wafting breeze of the rotting coffee. So had cases Foulke and Hodge had treated—a blacksmith's apprentice worked at Race and Water streets; the wife of a fisherman became infected by "sailing near the pestilential wharf." Rush thought back to his student days, thirty years earlier, when another ship offloaded rotting coffee just before the city's last major yellow fever epidemic erupted. It all, every single indicator Rush was hoping to find, slid into his brain at once. He looked at his two colleagues, never more certain of anything in his medical career: This, Rush told them, all pointed to bilious remitting yellow fever.[89]

The public mocked Rush mercilessly in the coming days as a frightened alarmist whose worry could wreck the city's trade. But about the fever's existence, Rush was right. As for where it came from or how to treat it, the famous doctor was miles off the mark. And that would cost lives and change the destiny of America's cities for the next one hundred years.

RUSH STAUNCHLY believed in something called miasma theory. The concept went back to the Roman Empire, possibly to Hippocrates himself. The basic idea of miasma theory is this: Things that stink cause disease. More specifically, the stink emits the seeds of disease into the atmosphere, people breathe it, and they get sick.[90] Here's why all this became so critical: Because of Rush and the swagger of his name, miasma theory emanated from Philadelphia's 1793 outbreak, confounding cities trying to defend themselves from disease for the next century.

The fever that year wrought more devastation than any yellow fever epidemic up to that time, and it happened in the country's most important city. Philadelphia was the nation's capital, and its largest city, with fifty thousand people. The University of Pennsylvania School of Medicine had been the nation's first and only medical school in the thirteen colonies, which made Philadelphia the focal point of the country's scientific thought.

Yellow fever slammed the door on all of that for ninety days that summer and fall. More than four thousand dead were officially reported, and everyone knew someone taken by the fever not on the official list. Most estimated that more than five thousand died. President George Washington fled the city. Vice President Thomas Jefferson evacuated to Monticello. Treasury Secretary Alexander Hamilton remained in the city, came down with the fever, and survived. That one summer muffled the city's progress. By 1800, Philadelphia's population had dropped to forty thousand. Yellow fever cleared the way for New York to become the nation's commercial center.

The destruction had other consequences: It created a massive stage for those who debated its causes. For decades after, doctors and nonmedical writers published tens of thousands of pages dissecting the epidemic. It was like an autopsy for an entire city, conducted in public.

Many Philadelphians, American doctors, European doctors, and others disagreed with Rush and the miasma theory. They believed in contagion. Contagion didn't fully mean what contagion means today, that a sick person is contagious and passes the illness on to others. The thinking behind contagionism was that the seeds of the virus had come from somewhere else, like a ship arriving in harbor. It was really an argument over whether the cause of a disease was local or imported.

Even sixty years later, in New Orleans, in Savannah and Charleston, in Norfolk and Portsmouth, most of the defensive tactics attempted after yellow fever broke out emerged from Philadelphia in 1793. To improve cleanliness, they paved their streets and sloped them to drain into the river. To ward off the chance of foul marsh "effluvia" producing gases that caused the fever, they filled low-lying tidal wetlands with wrecked boats, torn-down barns, destroyed piers, and loads of muck and dirt. They dispatched "scavengers," garbage collectors with carts, to remove detritus from the streets and gutters. And though sanitation was sorely needed in every American city, it wasn't the fix.

By the time 1793 rolled around, a slave uprising in Saint-Domingue, later Haiti, had been underway for nearly two years. Saint-Domingue reigned for much of the 1700s as a tiny part of an island that provided France with massive colonial wealth from its production of coffee, indigo, and sugar thanks to ease of shipping access to the growing American colonies. A sugar plantation owner didn't need vast business acumen to succeed. Since he paid no wages, big profits came easily. Saint-Domingue, though large by Caribbean standards, covers only eleven thousand square miles, the size of Maryland, yet every year imported as many as forty thousand enslaved Africans. So many of them died of yellow fever, malaria, and brutal beatings by planters that the abductions from Africa continued for decades to resupply their free-labor pool. The French colonists in Saint-Domingue drove as much as one-third of the Atlantic slave trade.[91]

By the late 1700s, nearly half a million slaves worked on the sugar and coffee plantations of Saint-Domingue, lorded over by just thirty thousand White, mostly French, colonials. Following its own revolution, the French National Assembly had approved the Declaration of the Rights of Man, which in law gave thousands of Blacks in the colony their freedom—except the White planters refused to allow it. On August 22, 1791, the slaves of Saint-Domingue rose up against their colonial rulers and the French colony plunged into a decade-long revolution.

In a desperate measure to restore peace, France declared an end to slavery as of August 29, 1793. It served little purpose; the rebels were already no longer enslaved, but the White planters continued to turn their heads from the law. The fallout from the 1793 deadline terrified the colonists on Saint-Domingue. As the date neared, thousands of Whites packed up their belongings, including their enslaved, and boarded ships for the United States to escape the chaos of revolution, to head to a place where they could still own other people. All that summer, ship after ship, their journey ended at Philadelphia's crowded waterfront.

IMMEDIATELY AFTER learning of the decaying coffee, Rush did what he did best. He did what only he and a few other doctors would have had the credibility, connections, or chutzpah to do. He went straight to the mayor. Matthew Clarkson, sixty years old, had a social standing and grace under pressure that made him tough to rattle. He had practiced surveying and engineering, was respected in mathematics and astronomy, and later helped found the Bank of Pennsylvania. Some thought Clarkson had developed his steadiness in business and political life through the school of hard knocks—though wealthy in his youth, he was orphaned at a young age and had to make his own way. He went to sea as a ship hand at age eight. His first job was as a clerk in one of Philadelphia's merchant trade houses. Or perhaps Clarkson's poise was born from the juxtaposition of his work against his home life, where he and his wife had nine children.[92]

Unlike Clarkson, Rush did not maintain an even temperament. He had been jacked up on adrenaline since he'd discovered the epidemic's cause. Rush told Clarkson that the seeds of this strange disease were transported by decaying miasma. It stemmed from filth in the city, on the streets, and in the air. A debate had raged for decades about whether epidemics such as yellow fever, typhoid, or cholera were caused by "dirty streets or dirty foreigners." It was easy for Rush to point out with disgust the rotting vegetables and decaying meat piled at the edge of streets. It didn't take a scientist to see the filth. A writer in the *Philadelphia Daily Advertiser* described the results:

"THE PRACTICE is to put the offals consisting of bones, with some flesh on them, the entrails of poultry, and many other corruptive matters in a barrel, in the yard, in some cases in cellars, where they putrify, and are very offensive, and must infect the air with a nauseous destructive quality, and I think less injury would probably follow from throwing them at once into the street, where the dogs would devour the meat, and the cows the vegetables."[93]

Clarkson didn't dispute Rush on sanitation nor that something deadly had infiltrated the city and that they had to find a way to tamp it down. Three days after Rush and the other doctors consulted down by Water Street, the papers quoted Clarkson saying that there was "great reason to apprehend that a dangerous, infectious disorder" had crept into the city. He summoned the scavengers to empty and clean the streets and gutters throughout town. Clarkson also had the newspapers print a reminder of a longstanding and often-ignored regulation: Residents must clean the walks in front of their houses, wash out their gutters, and pile their garbage on the streets on Mondays and Thursdays so the scavengers could haul it off.

But Clarkson also was a man of logic, of thoughtful science, and the value of approaching problems from many angles. He read the papers himself, talked to people, and knew to both highly respect Rush's medical theories as well as to take them with a shaker full of salt. He knew that many doctors in Philadelphia disagreed with Rush and were convinced that scourges like yellow fever were imported by either sick people or something that escaped through the bilge water or foul air of ships. Clarkson wanted a second opinion, a big one. He summoned the twenty-six fellows of the University of Pennsylvania College of Physicians, which included both Rush and his protégés as well as men like Doctor James Hutchinson, the city's port physician. Hutchinson didn't care for Rush. He often seemed to determine his own opinion merely by taking the opposite stance of Rush.

At the first meeting, ten of the members didn't show up. The sixteen esteemed fellows who attended agreed on one thing: that a debilitating and deadly disease had seeped into the city. That's it. Everything else was up for never-ending debate. Four men, including Rush, were appointed to a committee that was to file a report for consideration the next day. The committee agreed Rush could pen the draft. Rush went home and wrote well into the night. His report didn't use the words "yellow fever" nor did it settle the argument over whether the cause of the percolating epidemic was local or had come from afar. The report was a largely hollow salve, with the College of

Physicians going along with most of it. They recommended eleven measures for protection.[94] Most implied that the spread of the disease resulted from bad air:

"AVOID EVERY infected person, as much as possible.
Avoid fatigue of body and mind. Don't stand or sit in a draft, or in the sun, or in the evening air.
Dress according to the weather. Avoid intemperance. Drink sparingly of wine, beer, or cider.
When visiting the sick, use vinegar or camphor on your handkerchief, carry it in smelling bottles, use it frequently. Somehow mark every house with sickness in it, on the door or window.
Place your patients in the center of your biggest, airiest room, in beds without curtains. Change their clothes and bed linen often.
Stop the tolling of the bells at once." (Church bells had been ringing, to denote each death, and the physicians agreed that it was demoralizing the residents.)
"Bury the dead in closed carriages, as privately as possible. Clean the streets and keep them clean.
Stop building fires in your houses, or on the streets. They have no useful effect. But burn gunpowder. It clears the air. Most important of all, let a large and airy hospital be provided near the city, to receive poor people stricken with the disease who cannot otherwise be cared for."

This was their last chance to corral the spread, and that was it: Those actions were all the guidance that the most prominent group of medical minds in the country could muster. The committee didn't mention the influx of Saint-Domingue refugees. The port officer, Hutchinson, didn't cite the refugees either when he sent a requested report to the governor of Pennsylvania. He pointed out that another doctor had treated victims of the outbreak in a different part of the city, before the first cases on Water Street, which would have meant the illnesses had not originated with the rotting coffee. Hutchinson told the governor: "It does not appear to be an imported disease." He estimated there had been forty deaths. Rush, who unlike the port officer had been treating the victims himself, said it was more like one hundred fifty. Regardless of who was more accurate, the dying was only beginning.

On August 29, Rush wrote to his wife, Julia, who had taken their children and fled for safety, that he had never seen anything like the fever that now tromped through the city. The virus's symptoms, he said, vary from person to person: Sometimes, a victim is hit first with a fever and chills; more often, it sneaks in with a headache, upset stomach, and all-consuming fatigue:

> "THESE SYMPTOMS are followed by stupor, delirium, vomiting, a dry skin, cool or cold hands and feet, a feeble slow pulse . . . the eyes are at first diffused with blood, they afterwards become yellow, and in most cases a yellowness covers the whole skin on the third or fourth days. Few survive the fifth day, but more die on the second and third days . . . a bleeding at the nose, from the gums, and a vomiting of black matter in some instances close the scenes of life."[95]

All the typical remedies for fevers had failed, he told her. Bark, wine, and blisters didn't help. Hot vinegar soaked in blankets and laid over the patient did nothing. Occasionally, a cold bath had saved some, but not many. Rush was frustrated. "I have advised all the families that I attend that can move to quit the city. There is but one preventative that is certain, and that is to fly from it." Philadelphians did just that: fled town. By September, it seemed like the only ones left were the sick, the doctors, nurses, and ministers who stayed behind to tend to them, and the poor or the Black people who had no way out.

Rush and other doctors were already overwhelmed. He was distraught with his lack of success in treating patients. He wrote to his wife again: "You can recollect how much the loss of a single patient once a month used to affect me. Judge then how I must feel in hearing every morning about the death of three or four!" By September 1, Rush told her that thirty-eight people in eleven families had died in the past week on Water Street, location of the first cases, and many others throughout the city. Worse yet, he thought the fever had only begun its spread.

But a couple of days later, Rush's spirits were lifted by a treatment he was pioneering. He had begun prescribing calomel, which made people vomit, along with a dose of jalap, a drug derived from a root vegetable that worked as a laxative. He said patients' livers were often inflamed, and the purging caused them to expel the source of the irritation. Out of one hundred patients to whom Rush administered this treatment on the first day of their illness, none died, he said. "Some of my brethren rail at my new remedy," he wrote to Julia, "but they have seen little of the disease, and some of them not a single patient. Most of the publications come from those gentlemen. The new medicine bears down nearly all opposition. The deaths which now occur are chiefly poor people who have no doctors, or of respectable people who are in the hands of quacks or of the enemies of mercury." [96]

By the end of September, fourteen hundred Philadelphians were dead. The streets were empty. Burials were quick and without family, because no one knew if the virus could transmit from the air that surrounded a dead body. As October arrived, the virus grabbed an even more destructive gear. The daily death toll hit seventy, then eighty, then well over one hundred people, including entire families gone from earth at once. It was a devastating blow for Philadelphia. And in a young country still fighting for its existence, still pioneering life in its most important cities, it sent chills that rippled up and down the East Coast and the Mississippi. If this is what a visitation of yellow fever could wreak in the nation's capital, the nation's medical center, what would happen if it slammed relative outposts like Savannah, Charleston, New Orleans, or Norfolk? That's why, even before the city had recovered, the arguing began.

Philadelphians were still dying that fall when an Irish-born publisher named Matthew Carey, who had befriended Benjamin Franklin overseas and moved to Philadelphia, published a book on the epidemic: *A Short Account of the Malignant Fever, Lately Prevalent in Philadelphia*. People snapped it up—locals because it was about their city and those outside because they had to read every word of the recounting to even believe what happened. Nine days later, Carey put out a second edition, and in updates that followed he began including a list of deaths. Carey counted, with peoples' names listed right there on pages readers could touch, underline, and earmark, four thousand forty-four dead.[97] By nature of his prolific production line of new editions, with more information each time, the book became more than "A Short Account," it became the official record. What it did not become was the last word. Carey covered the "who and what" of the epidemic; disputes over the "why and how" took on a fevered fight of their own. And the arguing lasted for decades.

What really lit the fuse was a medical paper by a man named Colin Chisholm, a surgeon for the British artillery in Grenada in 1792 and 1793 when yellow fever broke out across the island. On July 10, 1795, the *Philadelphia Gazette* and *Universal Daily Advertiser* published the piece by Chisholm, a new work with "facts so highly interesting to the citizens of Philadelphia." It was Chisholm's account, *An Essay on the Malignant Pestilential Fever Introduced into the West Indie Islands*, his indisputable firsthand observations while treating patients.[98] For the American doctors who espoused the filthy-cities-local-origin theory of yellow fever, the title alone was asking for a fight. Introduced? That meant it came from somewhere else and somehow moved around. What about effluvia, miasma, bad air, malaria?

Chisholm's report attributed the yellow fever explosion in Grenada that summer to the arrival of a ship, the *Hankey*. That ship was full of two hundred seventy-five English settlers who had hoped to establish a colony on an island off the coast of Africa near Guinea, a place Chisholm called "Boullem," or Bolama Island. He wrote that the locals there were "ferocious to an extraordinary degree," so the settlers could not get off the ship and remained marooned on it just offshore for nine months.

"The rainy season coming on almost immediately after their arrival, and the heat being at the same time excessively great, they endeavored to shelter themselves from both, by raising the sides of the ship several feet, and covering her with a wooden roof," he wrote.

They abandoned any idea of a settlement, eventually sailing for Grenada, with the ship brewing a yellow fever transmission cycle along the way. Then Chisholm traced the route of the *Hankey* after it sailed from Grenada and reported that the fever had broken out at each stop, in Jamaica, in Saint-Domingue, and yes, in Philadelphia that summer of 1793. Residents of all American cities had a life-or-death interest in yellow fever, and publications along the East Coast ran excerpts of Chisholm's work for the next decade: The *Connecticut Courant* and the *Boston Gazette*, the *New York Evening Post*, the *New York Herald*, the *Philadelphia Daily Advertiser*, and many others.[99] It was as if Chisholm had insulted Rush's mother. Rush considered it a rash of well-distributed impertinent information. Neither he nor his legion of protégés would sit by for such effrontery.

Rush placed himself among a cluster of medical writers who argued that, because yellow fever sprang up due to local causes, the only people who could theorize about those causes were those with firsthand experience. If yellow fever was an American plague, only American doctors and medical writers should be espousing theories about it. Rush's friend Noah Webster couldn't have agreed more. Webster, a lawyer, educator, farmer, eventually an epidemiologist, and a proud nationalist, had become well-known for his linguistic work. In 1783, he published *A Grammatical Institute of the English Language*, a three-part work that opened with a "speller" that prescribed how Americans should spell many words differently than in British English: "Our political harmony is therefore conceived in a uniformity of language." He would eventually iterate this work into a full-fledged dictionary intended to unite the young country around its own version of the language. With a series of East Coast yellow fever epidemics choking commercial trade for much of the 1790s, Webster didn't hesitate to extend his America-first, American-only work into the raging fight over whether yellow fever was local or imported. He penned a letter to Rush in December 1798 lambasting the Philadelphians who had petitioned Congress to ban the arrival of ships from the West Indies and the Mediterranean during the summer:

> "THIS PROPOSITION is something worse than folly. It is a serious attack on the commercial interests of this country. I can ascribe it only to insanity, for you are sensible that madness is often epidemic after pestilence."

Webster and Rush also were involved in another publication venture, a clever Trojan horse for their cultural agenda. *The Medical Repository* entered the fray in 1797. Conceived by Elihu Hubbard Smith, Edward Miller, and Samuel L. Mitchell, the *Repository's* mission was to fill a void for American-written medical publications. Smith and Miller had been understudies of Rush during medical school in Philadelphia, and in their first edition, they explained that the *Repository* had particular interest in improving understanding of disease, notably yellow fever. They told their readers that American doctors and even medical writers who were not doctors, like Webster, had the scientific advantage of being present during outbreaks with "the opportunities it affords" to document and compare the diseases. The theory of contagion, that a fever could be imported on a ship, was based on "book knowledge."[100]

When the man who edited the medical section of *Encyclopedia Britannica* published a paper on yellow fever, the *Repository* shot it down. James Tyler, the editor, had not personally experienced plagues and pestilence, and the editors told him he was not "entitled to the character of an original observer of events and occurrences, in such time of public commotion."

The Medical Repository editors made no effort to contain their snark when a diplomat in Marseilles, France, at the request of Secretary of State James Madison, wrote to convey ideas about containing disease outbreaks. Marseilles had been devastated during several waves of the bubonic plague, including in 1720 when it killed one hundred thousand people. "Our readers will smile to learn," the editors of the *Repository* wrote, "that they propose to destroy the contagion by the burning of cascarilla and spruce (they perhaps mean pine) wood, and to prevent the operation of it by the smoking of tobacco and the application of cauteries."

Madison particularly wanted a report on the lazaretto, or quarantine station, that Marseille had established for incoming ships. The editors reserved their sharpest sarcasm for that suggestion: "The Consul refers to the regulations of their lazaretto for information as to the method of stopping the contagion, which they seem to think are effectual there, and, of course, must be infallible in all other places."

With the easy pickings taken care of, *Repository* editors then rotated the barrels of their cannons to their biggest problem, British doctor Chisholm and his essay on fever in the West Indies. Chisholm's piece had become a dark cloud, blocking the light from their most important writings and concepts. His work seemed to have it all: firsthand case studies and observations, detailed documentation of the local climate down to daily wind and temperature readings, and Chisholm's long residence on the island. The *Repository* editors spared no paper and ink for the necessary beat-down. They turned over nearly the entire edition of the journal to Webster and Smith, who teamed up to pen a twenty-five-page review, undoubtedly with Rush on ghost-writing

duty. Webster and Smith were opposed to slavery, and they homed in
on Chisholm's role as a participant in the slave trade, as an owner of
a plantation on Grenada.[101] They noted that the original passengers
on the ship *Hankey* had gone to Bolama on a mission to establish a
settlement on the African continent where slavery was illegal.

Rush and Webster were not the least impressed with Chisholm's
fastidious accounts of the daily weather; in fact, they noted, the tables
matched the observations they and others had made about the climatic
effects of weather on illness in the United States—all of which, they
said, proved instead of disproved their theory that local conditions
create the foul air in which yellow fever and nearly all other diseases
incubate. In case the critique by Rush and Webster wasn't enough,
afterward the *Repository* sought out pieces by other West Indies-based
writers to "correct" Chisholm's work.

Though the *Repository* editors, along with Rush and Webster, may
have thought they had settled the issue, Chisholm's work had many
defenders. Chisholm and his advocates would deliver speeches and
publish articles in England or France aimed at one audience: Rush,
Webster, and their followers. It was Revolutionary-era trolling.

The ongoing dispute had a horrendous result for American cities
along the East Coast. Those cities seemed to be taking turns getting
decimated by yellow fever, and they had no idea how to stop it. None
of the possibilities of the outbreak's sources had been eliminated. It
could stem from the marshes, rotting food, poor ventilation, swampy
streets, or it could come from ships.

Even sixty-plus years after Philadelphia's worst epidemic, when
Portsmouth's vice mayor and its health officer, Doctor Joseph Schoolfield,
sat down in that awful summer of 1855 to consider what actions to take
amid the fomenting epidemic, his view was that Rush was "the very best
authority in this disease." In a post-mortem on the fever's destruction
that Schoolfield penned on behalf of the town of Portsmouth, he leaned
on Rush. "The yellow fever is not derived from specific contagion; it is
always generated by putrefaction," Schoolfield noted, quoting Rush. "It

is not, and while the laws of nature retain their present order, never can be imported so as to become an epidemic in any country."[102]

Schoolfield, and all the residents of the Virginia port cities, were about to become a case study in just how deadly bad information could be.

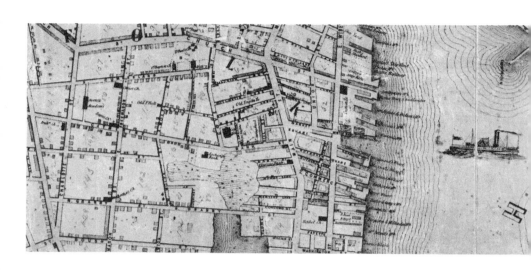

The central part of Norfolk, Virginia, with its wharves jutting into the Elizabeth River, from James Keily's 1851 map.

CHAPTER SEVEN
TRAPPED

SADNESS dripped from the letter Winchester Watts wrote his brother on August 5. Matter-of-fact declarations laid bare his isolation. Watts, president of the Portsmouth Common Council, found himself almost running the town alone.

"Nearly all businesses closed their stores yesterday afternoon," Watts wrote to his brother, Samuel. "Only two groceries were kept open. Several of the council are sick, and others have left, and we are without a quorum. No money can be obtained at the bank. There is no decline of the fever."

The night before, Watts left Portsmouth briefly to help his sister and two friends evacuate to Old Point Comfort, but as they approached the Point, a steamer pulled up beside them. The commanding officer at Old Point had issued orders prohibiting any boats from Norfolk or Portsmouth from landing.[103] Watts returned home, and his sister and her friends took a second steamer to Baltimore instead.

Watts had committed to staying in Portsmouth yet now stared down what that really meant. It would be a life of survivalism, and even that didn't factor in trying to avoid the fever. He'd have to stock up on food, so he laid in a supply of ducks and chickens. He knew that he'd have to parse his cash because the bank had already given out more money than it had in deposits. For all practical purposes, he was the Town Council. He'd make all the decisions, take all the actions, and assume all responsibility for anything that went wrong. On top of that, all his friends had fled.

Among all other things, Watts was now also responsible for taking the donations that had begun to come in from people around the country, converting it to whatever the residents needed most and acknowledging the contribution with a return letter. A letter from a man in Staunton, Virginia, had arrived that morning with a one hundred dollar check to help the sick and starving.

Watts felt alone and trapped. After his sister and friends were repelled from Old Point Comfort, he heard of several Portsmouth residents who tried to get out of town to the west—the only direction not locked in by water. As soon as people in neighboring Suffolk discovered the refugees, they called a town meeting and evicted the Portsmouth family. Another man and his family, who didn't know of the other cities' quarantines, were turned back at the wharf from boarding a steamer bound for Baltimore.[104] "Are we supposed to stay in Gosport and die?" he asked, then sat down on the pier and cried. But determined to get his family out of town, he rented a wagon and they headed to the house of acquaintances who had agreed to put them up. Once there, the host family became frightened. After about an hour, the Portsmouth refugees had to go back at night in the rain. A few days later, they finally caught a steamer to Philadelphia.

"The town looks dull and gloomy," Watts wrote, "and if I could consciously leave, I would be off without delay."

Reverend James Chisholm, the Episcopal priest who had helped remove Irish from the Gosport tenements, watched civilization in Portsmouth crumble hour by hour. A sick German husband and wife and their daughter were carried from their house to the hospital cart by the doctor and priest. "No other aid could be obtained," Chisholm noted, "even though the opposite pavement was crowded with curious spectators." The family's two little boys sat outside and stared blankly.

The town had not made provisions for orphans, and when the crowd dispersed, the boys remained in the house to fend for themselves.[105]

Few who were not living in the midst of the fever, such as Watts, knew how rapidly it was spreading, the way it had already blanketed the town in desolation, or even knew a reliable count of the dead and dying. Those reading the *Richmond Dispatch* on August 2 were told that Norfolk had only six new cases and no deaths and that the disease remained contained in Barry's Row. The paper reported six new cases and five deaths in Gosport and Portsmouth, which wouldn't explain the scarcity of coffins in town. Families had to order coffins ahead of time, even as loved ones fought to stay alive. Portsmouth was out of hospital beds for the sick. Watts wrote to President Franklin Pierce and asked permission to use the Naval Hospital in Portsmouth. Pierce and the secretary of the Navy granted access to one wing. Yet, it was tough to find nurses willing to tend to yellow fever victims despite the general agreement that the sick could not infect those around them. It was even hard to find carriage drivers to haul those ailing to the hospital.

Despite all that, the *Southern Argus*, a Norfolk paper with Know Nothing sympathies, saw nothing to fear in its report on August 4:

> "WE ANNOUNCE with much pleasure, that the fever seems to have spent itself in Barry's Row, and upon some of the hapless residents of those damp, filthy and unventilated tenements ... The few who are sick, or most of them, are rapidly recovering under skillful treatment, and it is sincerely hoped that in a few days we shall have the happiness to declare every part of Norfolk entirely free of epidemic disease."

The *Argus*, of course, would never experience the happiness of declaring Norfolk free of epidemic disease, at least that summer. And it was in good company in sloughing off the threat of disease imported by ships. As Norfolk and Portsmouth residents either fled town or bunkered in, arguments raged about quarantine precautions.

The debate sprung from a quarantine law put in place in New Orleans that summer. Though it had taken a deadly punch two years earlier, New Orleans again confronted a yellow fever outbreak in 1855. Governor Paul O. Herbert and the legislature were determined to quash it to avoid a repeat of the 1853 epidemic that had killed nearly eight thousand people. They enacted a ten-day quarantine for any ship coming into New Orleans from an infected port.[106] The governor then issued another proclamation naming Veracruz, San Juan de Nicaragua, and Havana infected.[107] Ship captains tested the law immediately by "running quarantine."

The captain of the *Crescent City* steamed from Havana to the New Orleans harbor and simply refused to stop at quarantine. He had a load of cargo and would have to depart for New York in five days. He had made a financial decision: He chose to pay a two thousand dollar fine, thus sparing the shipping line many more thousands in lost time and spoiled fruit and coffee.

A *New York Times* correspondent wrote that these were unfortunate circumstances for the shipping line yet vastly more unfortunate for New Orleans. If enforced, the quarantine would effectively shut down the city as a shipping hub every summer for six months. The long delay at quarantine, or the elimination of Havana as a weigh station, would render most shipping lines through New Orleans money losers. Think about it, the *Times* wrote: Could a shipper turn a profit if a steamer had to spend ten days in quarantine at Havana, ten days in quarantine in New Orleans, all for a twelve-day out-and-back route?

The answer was "no" from the New York owners of a line of steamers. They wrote their agent in New Orleans asking if the *Crescent City* had been quarantined or if the *Grenada* would be quarantined in New Orleans. The *Grenada* had to touch in Havana because it was a relay for mail from California. The Board of Health confirmed that both would be subject to the ten-day hold in quarantine.

New Orleans appeared to be erupting again with yellow fever despite the efforts to quell the outbreak. The *New Orleans Bee*, formerly a Whig and now a Know Nothing paper, lashed out. "Of all ridiculous and nonsensical enactments, this Quarantine is the most stupendous," the *Bee* wrote. "The law should be called an act to harass, impede, shackle and injure the commerce and navigation of New Orleans."

The *Bee* predicted that if the restrictions were not lifted in the next couple of weeks, the California line of steamers and the Mexico line would abandon their New Orleans routes. The *Bee's* outrage stemmed from the "unmeaning and senseless clamor raised by certain parties" that yellow fever originated in foreign ports rather than locally.[108] Sixty years after the 1793 epidemic in Philadelphia, when Benjamin Rush and Noah Webster published tens of thousands of words arguing that yellow fever erupted from local causes, their errant theory still fueled the argument of the commerce-above-all-else crowd that wanted to keep businesses open.

Considering the need for yet another quarantine of New Orleans, the *New York Times* penned an obituary for the Gulf Coast city:

"WE HAVE HAD occasion before to exhibit the folly of attempting to bring New Orleans into the field, as a rival of New York, for the trade of the West. The climate and sensitive health of the place forbid the idea . . . New Orleans must presently pass from the list of great sea-ports and depots. It will be obliged to withdraw from active business, in consequence of ill-health."[109]

The *Times* changed its tune a month later, when the threat of yellow fever erupted in Norfolk. Perhaps it had to do with the 1,681-nautical-mile buffer between New Orleans and New York versus the quick three-hundred-fifty-mile sail from Norfolk. New York was among the first cities to proclaim a quarantine against ships from Norfolk, subjecting them to a thirty-day wait on the Hudson before landing at a wharf. Steamers from the infected Virginia ports quickly developed tactics to dodge the quarantine by loading passengers, luggage, and cargo at a landing five miles outside the cities, allowing the captain to say the ship had not touched in Norfolk or Portsmouth.

"Is there no remedy of protection?" the *Times* asked. "If there is, it should be resorted to immediately, before the City of New York becomes as bad off from the scourge of yellow fever as is Norfolk, Portsmouth and Gosport. Or if not, then let the quarantine be abolished, as a humbug and useless clog upon commerce."

On Tuesday, August 7, thirty-eight days after Doctor John Trugien treated the first cases of yellow fever in Gosport, Reverend George Armstrong felt upbeat. It was a clear, bright morning as he strode through the center of Norfolk, down Church Street to the National Hotel, right onto Main past the fire company and through Market Square, toward the Ferry Wharf. He was headed across the river to Portsmouth to check on a minister friend who he'd heard had been stricken with the fever.

Armstrong could see that Norfolk didn't have its usual bustle that morning, and that made sense because about half the population had fled during that first week of August. Yet everything seemed cheerful. He figured a visitor to Norfolk, unaware of how busy it usually was, wouldn't notice anything to suggest that yellow fever had taken root in the city. He felt more optimistic than he had in several days because, for one thing, the Board of Health that morning reported "no deaths" the day before. One man he chatted with on the way through town said he was enjoying the city more now, with less commotion. "Now that the more excitable portion of our people have fled," he told Armstrong, "we shall have a quiet time again."

Forty-one-year-old Armstrong, a smallish, spry man, was a well-known sight downtown. Each day, he looped through the streets and alleys to visit church members and chatted with other ministers, city leaders, or anyone else he ran into. He continued his trek that August morning toward the Norfolk wharf. Waiting on the ferry pier, he could clearly see the ships anchored on the other side and even Portsmouth's buildings beyond the shipyards. But Armstrong had not walked the streets of Portsmouth in more than a week. He'd only heard talk of the fever's spread—mostly rumors, he figured, from frightened people.

Armstrong read several local newspapers every day, but they had not been painting a real picture of the fever's advancement. Several editors and compositors at Portsmouth's three daily papers had already become sick. They struggled to keep the presses running. The instant delivery of information by telegraph between Norfolk and Richmond had ceased: The operator of the telegraph had abandoned his job to get himself and his family out of the city. That delayed the gathering and sending of eyewitness information to the outside world.

The moment Armstrong stepped off the ferry in Portsmouth, he stopped in his tracks. An apocalyptic scene lay before him. A haze clouded the air, smoked up by the barrels of tar that residents lit to keep the "bad air" away. A white hue colored everything on the ground, from the barrel after barrel of lime the people had spread around to disinfect. The fleeing residents had dumped food, entrails, leftover milk, and anything and everything else that was perishable at the edge of their properties. It hadn't rained since the mass exodus, so the detritus lay rotting in the summer sun. The streets were nearly deserted.

Armstrong walked through the haze in disbelief. He paused again at the city market, usually crowded with people who'd driven carts from the country to sell produce. He saw only two carts. "Drivers of these carts were sitting on the curbstone beside them, and they, with their horses, looked as if wilted down by the heat," he wrote, "and I saw no one there present to buy their marketing."[110]

He covered half the length of the commercial district in Portsmouth to get to his friend's house. He only saw one other person and one open store. A voracious reader, a letter writer and correspondent with educated men throughout the East Coast, he'd read many times about yellow fever. But for the first time, he saw with his own eyes the damage that would happen should the fever get a footing in Norfolk. *What on Earth had happened in Portsmouth?* he wondered. *How could a place change this much in just one week?*

From Armstrong's outward appearance, he seemed a mild-mannered minister who took things as they came. He was not. Though he presented his opinions as the result of studious debate, only determined after long and eloquent consideration, he'd take a stand and dare all-comers to push him off it. He looked around and thought other cities' quarantines were unenforceable and mean-spirited and created needless problems. He knew the virus was spreading, and he and his wife had talked about that when they debated whether to stay in town. But he supported others fleeing and had a personal experience to conclude that the refugees wouldn't transport the virus to other places. "I well recollect, although then a child, that in 1822 when fever prevailed in New York City, great numbers of the inhabitants of the city came out to Bloomfield, New Jersey, where I was then living; and one at the most died of the fever there, and yet no case originated in the village."

The panic, Armstrong decided, was more due to the quarantine regulations and the possibility of being trapped than the threat of getting sick from the virus. A vast transportation web stretched from state to state by 1855—rail lines across the land, steamships via the ocean, rivers, and bays. To cut off all communication and travel effectively "in a country like ours is an impossibility," he thought. He chuckled at how the locals had initially foiled Baltimore's quarantine: Residents would take a boat for the Eastern Shore in the morning and return on the same boat in the afternoon, as if they lived on the Shore, then board the boat to Baltimore. He appreciated that Virginia Governor Henry Wise had not only kept the boats running back and forth but opened his own Eastern Shore property to refugees. He even added more outhouses.

Things were different down in North Carolina, Armstrong had read. The town of Weldon enacted an ordinance that banned anyone who had been in Norfolk or Portsmouth in the past fifteen days from setting foot in the village. If they were White, they'd face a fine of one hundred dollars a day. If the person was enslaved or free and Black, the penalty was "nine-and-thirty lashes on his bare back." In his journal, Armstrong translated that with irony: "That is, in substance, if any poor negro, likely to have fever in their blood, shall enter our town of Weldon we'll strip to the skin and lay the lash, and then turn the fugitive out into the swamps to die. Terror must have driven the people of Weldon mad when they adopted such an order as this."

As Armstrong left his minister friend's house that Tuesday in Portsmouth, all this swirled in his mind. On his way back to the ferry, he weaved through different streets in town. The air swirled with bruise-colored tar smoke. Entire blocks had been abandoned. Dogs and chickens scrounged for scraps in the yards of empty houses. He paused to watch a man knock at the front door of a house and a woman leaning out of an upper window to respond to him. Armstrong thought she looked frightened to even be that close to the man. At the ferry house, he chatted with several Portsmouth residents. The only topic? Which of their friends was sick and who had died.

"I've taken seven orders for coffins already today," an undertaker told Armstrong.

The strangest thing, though, wasn't what Armstrong saw. It was what he heard. Normally, by 10 a.m. on a weekday, in a shipbuilding town like Portsmouth, the air would be filled with the cacophony of workers hammering and sawing and shouting and the clamor of cartwheels and horse hooves clattering over cobblestone streets. He would have heard children playing, vendors calling out to hawk fruits and vegetables. There was none of that. The only thing Armstrong heard was a rooster's lonesome echo.

His optimism of three hours earlier had turned to dread. "Never before have I had as lively a conception of the utter desolation of a plague-stricken city," he wrote that day. "Portsmouth presents the most deserted, forlorn appearance of any place I have ever seen."

Norfolk, he now thought, could not be far behind.

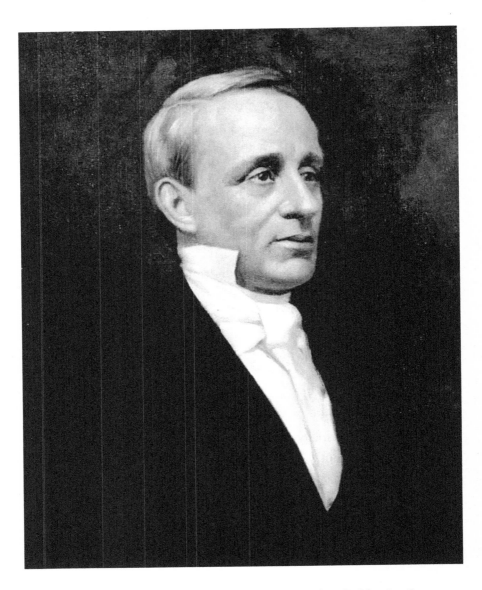

Reverend George Armstrong, courtesy of Walter B. Martin, Jr., Armstrong's great-grandson, via USGenWeb.

CHAPTER EIGHT

VENGEANCE

THE evening after returning from seeing the devastation in Portsmouth, George Armstrong was eating dinner with his family when fire bells began clanging. He jumped up from the table and raced to the front door to see smoke rising several blocks away. Immediately, he suspected he knew what was on fire: Barry's Row. His stomach sank.

Fires in a city full of wood-framed houses, barns, ships, and wharves were common, and Armstrong didn't go to most of them. In this case, an indigent woman from his congregation lived nearby and he wanted to see if she was okay. She was, but what he saw made him realize the people of his city were not. Flames engulfed the upper end of the twelve townhouses on Barry's Row. He guessed more than three thousand people stood around watching the show, not just transfixed by the flames but cheering on the destruction.

"The fire companies had their engines all there to protect the houses around," Armstrong noted, "but not a drop of water were they attempting to throw upon the burning buildings."[111]

The *Norfolk Beacon*, along with the *Southern Argus*, had been scapegoating Barry's Row for weeks as the spark of all yellow fever infections in Norfolk. Just three days earlier, the *Beacon* reported that as evidence of the "crowded state" at Barry's Row, sixteen Irish workers slept in just one room of an apartment. Along with the landlord's family, at least thirty people shared the house.

The townspeople, though, were particularly angry with the owners of Barry's Row. After the city removed the sick to the makeshift hospital outside of town, officials evicted residents who were not sick and boarded up and fenced off the Row. Rumors flew that the owner of Barry's Row had surreptitiously rented the newly vacant apartments to people who had fled Irish Row in Gosport. Armstrong didn't know whether that rumor had credence because fears masked as facts had been flying all over town for weeks. Even if it was true, he didn't think it justified torching the buildings. He suspected many of the gleeful spectators would soon regret standing idly by and approving of "lawless violence."

"In the unprotected condition in which our city must soon be, if the fever should rage here as it is in Portsmouth now, none can tell the effect of such a precedent," he wrote.

No one would ever be pursued, let alone charged, with setting the fire. But an even bigger problem existed. Burning Barry's Row had not had the intended effect of slowing or stopping yellow fever's advancement throughout Norfolk. In fact, the virus seemed to be drifting much like the smoke from the fire, starting in one spot then wafting around town in the breeze.

No one knew how many were dying. The Norfolk Sanitary Committee, formed to track the spread, reported the day after the Barry's Row fire that no new infections and no deaths had "come to the attention of the board." In Portsmouth, the *Richmond Dispatch* reported that the fever was on the increase and more than half the residents had fled town. It summarized the situation across the river with no details: "The reports from Norfolk are truly alarming."

Armstrong tapped into his network of parishioners, doctors, friends, and newspaper correspondents and tallied up his own count on August 11. As best he could figure, Norfolk doctors had treated sixty cases so far and twenty of the victims had died.[112] That fatality rate would remain a person's odds throughout the epidemic. If someone caught the fever, he had a one out of three chance of dying.

Regardless of the lack of reliable numbers, or the newspapers' continued confidence that the fever was disappearing, all the things that people could see with their own eyes pointed to a mushrooming epidemic. The *Dispatch* reported that the steamer *Jamestown* arrived in Richmond with refugees from Norfolk who had somehow skirted the quarantine: "Passengers on the *Jamestown* report that the fever is much worse in Norfolk than represented either by the press or the Sanitary Committee."[113]

A Baltimore doctor riding the steamer *Louisiana* at the request of his city's Sanitary Committee arrived home the evening of August 7, reporting that Norfolk appeared to be entirely abandoned, the streets deserted, and stores closed, with people still fleeing in any direction they could go. The *Louisiana* had arrived that day with four hundred seventy-five Norfolk residents crammed on board. Two hundred of them were children, who slept on the floors of the steamer's saloons on the way up the Chesapeake Bay.

The newspapers began publishing an item every day titled "List of the Dead." On August 7, a *Dispatch* special edition reported devastating news for Portsmouth's ability to endure the epidemic: "J.N. Schoolfield, chairman of the Sanitary Committee, is dead." Doctor Schoolfield had coached the towns' residents through the epidemic to this point, and now the paper reported they were rudderless.

The following day, the *Petersburg Express* list read:

"WM. DUGAN; Mrs. Herald, wife of John Herald, deceased; Patrick Galilee; Jas. Fortune; Mrs. Mary Cooke; Alexander Godwin; Mrs. A. Godwin (These are the last of a family of twelve, every one of whom have been swept off with the fever during the past two weeks.) Mrs. Martin Flaherty, a most excellent woman; John Shannon, a youth, son of J.H.

Shannon; Mrs. Waters; Mrs. Daniel Sullivan; Mrs. O'Niel;
Robert Ash, son of William Ash; John K. Pendleton, a
most excellent young man and Captain's clerk on board
the U.S. Ship Pennsylvania; Nancy Higgs, a sister-in-law
of Geo. Marshall, deceased; Moses Quarles, an overseer
of the Navy Yard; Mrs. Brinkley Saunders; Mrs. Ayler,
a widow lady; Miss Brown, a young daughter of Wm. D.
Brown, ship carpenter. Making in all 20, which added to
those previously reported, number 66."

The blossoming number of deaths at the end of the first week of
August perfectly matched the timing of a weather-driven mosquito
eruption. At 2:30 in the afternoon on the last day of July, thunder and
lightning cracked the skies over Portsmouth and Norfolk. Reverend
James Chisholm, the Episcopal minister who had helped move the
sick from Irish Row in Gosport, wrote of a "very damp atmosphere,
with frequent showers all day long."[114] It hadn't rained a drop in the
previous two and a half weeks, then on July 31 the skies dumped
nearly half an inch of rain.[115]

Rain fell into wagon ruts, horse hoof indentations, sunken spots
in yards, and potholes in the streets and raised the water levels in
cisterns. It swamped mosquito eggs deposited by the hundreds on
dry ground, the emerging clusters bobbing unnoticed in puddles. In
hot summer weather, the eggs raced through their pupa and larva
phases.[116] Almost at once, right around August 8, swarms of adult
mosquitoes rose from the ground. When the females sought blood
meals to fortify their eggs, they attacked the nearest person.

Viruses need a host to live and spread. The yellow fever virus
now had two: the mosquitoes that carried it and the people infected
with it. The infected residents unknowingly transported the virus to
a new place wherever they moved around town. With the mosquito
population catalyzed by the July 31 storms, the number of infected
people and mosquitoes exploded.

The sick had not yet reached a catastrophic level, and Portsmouth could still either tend to most of its fever victims or transport them to the Naval Hospital. It was the same over in Norfolk, where the city could haul the sick to the old horse racing track nestled in a grove of live oaks. There, volunteer nurse Annie Andrews was working herself ragged tending to the sick, not to mention her efforts to repair the shabby buildings that people were calling a hospital.

Andrews had been the first volunteer nurse who newly elected Mayor Hunter Woodis brought to Julappi Hospital. The hospital consisted of one large run-down building, which Andrews called "a miserable house," along with three outbuildings. For a good while, its staff was just Andrews and the three Sisters of Charity from Emmitsburg, Maryland, who Andrews would only ever know by their first names: Sister Susannah cooked while Sisters Christine and Mary Levis tended to patients. The newspaper had announced Andrews's arrival by misnaming her "Lucy Andrews," and many thought she was one of the Catholic volunteers. Though Andrews was Protestant, the sisters jokingly nicknamed her "Sister Lucia," a term of endearment that caught on with patients.

Woodis felt personally responsible for the women he'd assigned to Julappi, so the mayor himself usually drove the wagon that carted the next batch of sick out there. Sometimes, on the four-mile wagon ride, a patient would become a corpse and would have to ride back into town with Woodis. Usually, Andrews figured she and the sisters tended sixty to seventy sick at a time. On a bad day, twenty or thirty patients died.

The July 31 thunderstorms sent streams of water pouring through the ceiling of the main building. Andrews climbed on the roof and caulked the seams. She caulked the ones in the walls, too, after water sluiced through them. After a few weeks, her hands wore thin and developed blisters. She wouldn't allow herself to stop working, so she soaked her hands in salt water until calluses formed.[117]

Work at the hospital was physically taxing and, at times, terrifying.

Woodis, Doctor George Upshur, and William Ferguson, president of the newly formed relief association in Norfolk, came and went often. But the women were the only ones who lived there day and night.

On one quiet night, Andrews and Sister Christine had the main building full of patients, with others spread among two of the smaller buildings. A man on a couch in one of the outbuildings moaned and wailed while the two nurses tended to a dying patient. A woman nearby shouted at the nurses: "Liquor, more liquor!" She became more frantic when they refused and began cursing them. "Sister Christine and Sister Lucia are both drunk!" she yelled.

Moments later, the nurses heard more "mournful wailing, sobbing, sighing, shrieking" from a pine thicket out in the dark woods. They had no patient that far from the building and decided it was a prankster trying to scare them. "I am not nervous, but this staggers me," Andrews thought. She decided she'd talk to Woodis the next day about assigning someone to the hospital for security.

Late that night, after the prankster had gone, Andrews walked outside of the main hospital toward the smaller building that she shared with the Sisters of Charity. She stood and looked up at the stars blanketing the sky. Moonlight glimmered off the broad Elizabeth River and the breeze hit her face. She saw the long, craggy arms of live oaks silhouetted against the dark. For a rare moment, Andrews stood and absorbed the calm.

All told, in Norfolk and Portsmouth, one hundred sixty people died of yellow fever from June 30, when Doctor John Trugien identified the first cases in Gosport, through August 15. Not all of them had to die. People didn't know if it was safe to tend to sick family and friends, so they kept away. Those who were well fled their homes, leaving the stricken to fend for themselves. Some died of starvation. In other cases, the human body could not continue to expel fluids without being replenished. Their organs, attacked by the virus, shut down due to dehydration.

Armstrong recounted a story that many of the people in both

cities heard about an Irish man named Stapleton. He rented a room in a family's house down by the river on the Norfolk side. After Stapleton came down with the fever, the landlord and his family brought him food and water for a day or two. Then they became terrified and fled. They left Stapleton in a room in the attic with no food or water. Even in a state of delirium, Stapleton figured out he'd been left alone. He got dressed and walked down the street toward a nearby doctor's office.

"His strength held out until he reached the door, and there he fell and died in the street," Armstrong wrote. "And what makes the case more sad is that he is said to have many friends at home, but here he was a stranger in a strange land."[118]

Unlike Stapleton, some yellow fever victims died because they refused treatment. Andrews had been at the Julappi Hospital for about three weeks when Woodis arrived one day. Would you mind going into town with me? the mayor asked Andrews. There's a family in desperate need of care.

They took a carriage into the city and were left waiting at the house for a good while before someone came to speak to them. The woman who greeted them, a family friend from out of town, said that they did not want or need nursing care. Andrews couldn't fathom that. The family was dying.

She is not prepared to receive visitors, the family friend said of the mother.

Andrews still didn't understand. "I was not there to be entertained," Andrews said.

The family friend insisted that no care was needed. Andrews and Woodis got back in the carriage. Along the way to Julappi, Woodis explained that they'd refused his help because he was Catholic, so he brought Andrews. But the family had assumed Andrews was "a Papist disguised." The family members were staunch, anti-Catholic Know Nothings. They'd sooner fend for themselves than be helped by a Catholic.[119]

To prevent situations like Stapleton's death, Woodis and Norfolk leaders formed a relief organization called the Howard Association on August 14 and named William Ferguson as president. The association began with three thousand dollars, an amount that would swell in coming weeks as more and more of the country's residents turned their attention toward the disaster in Virginia.

In a positive development, Doctor Joseph Schoolfield had recovered from his reported death. Schoolfield was sick, not dead. On August 9, Winchester Watts wrote to his brother, Samuel, saying that Schoolfield had been taken to the Naval Hospital. Two other Portsmouth doctors had also come down with the fever. The Naval Hospital also had taken in "a large number" of orphaned children, while Watts and others tried to secure a house and caretakers in town to convert to an orphanage.

Watts embraced his responsibilities. He was not just president of the Portsmouth Common Council but also president of the Portsmouth Savings Fund Society. And he ran a commercial icehouse that he and his brother owned. The bank's cashier, George Bain, showed up at the icehouse the morning of August 9. He wanted to flee to Richmond, to join his family who had been writing daily to implore him to get away. Watts said he didn't blame Bain.

A few ministers even fled. In times of crisis, with doctors becoming sick and nurses difficult to find, ministers became de facto nurses, checking on parishioners daily to hand them water, cover them with sheets, or offer calming words. Watts told his brother he had seen and heard acts of inhumanity he could not have comprehended before—men deserting their families, adult children abandoning their sick mothers and fathers. Schoolfield's wife did not forsake him, Watts wrote. "Dr. Schoolfield is quite sick. His wife goes to the hospital every day."

Watts had written to his brother daily since Samuel left for Richmond. It seemed as if his brother was his only connection to a normal world, one that had vanished before his eyes within a few weeks. He begged Samuel to write back daily. "The mail did not arrive until late last evening," he wrote one day. "I waited until it was opened, anticipating a letter from you, but none came and I was disappointed."

Relief funds started to arrive, and Watts spent most mornings writing letters to acknowledge the donations. Some of the money would go toward a house Watts had procured to convert to an orphanage for the more than thirty children now at the Naval Hospital. He'd have to arrange for food, clothing, bedding, and people to tend to them—and transportation from the hospital to the house. Of all things, he was concerned with how the town would be able to sustain itself financially: "The town will have a heavy bill to pay."

Samuel Watts told Winchester that he might relocate from Richmond to Baltimore, but Winchester told his brother to head to the mountains. He was convinced that the fever would spread to other coastal cities. Above all, stay away from Portsmouth, he said.

"The streets look solitary and desolate. Private dwellings are generally closed. Do not make yourself at all uneasy about me. I cannot leave here now. Write me every day."[120]

The outbreak had not directly hit George Armstrong, his family, or his church yet. Norfolk remained a week or two behind Portsmouth, so Armstrong donned his logical, scientific hat and pulled out some paper. He couldn't make sense of something his friend and parishioner, Doctor Upshur, had told him: Upshur had treated his first case of yellow fever on July 16. From what anyone knew, the first refugees from Irish Row in Gosport fled across the river to Norfolk four days after that. The fever, Armstrong deduced, must have been in Norfolk before the Gosport refugees arrived.

Armstrong began plotting the points where the fever first appeared.

Being well-read and interested in natural phenomena, Armstrong would have heard of Doctor John Snow's epidemiological work during the cholera outbreak in London the year before when six hundred sixteen people died. Snow had plotted the deaths and linked them to a public water pump. As soon as Snow removed the pump handle, the outbreak sputtered to an end.[121]

Armstrong began with three points on his map: Page and Allen's

Shipyard to the south; Fox's house on Scott's Creek to the northwest; and Barry's Row to the northeast. He drew a line between the three points, revealing a nearly equilateral triangle with about a mile and a half on each side. Then he looked at the weather readings taken daily at Fort Monroe and at Old Point Comfort and reported to the Army's surgeon general.

The weather report's daily readings showed that the breezes in June and July had prevailed from the south, pushing winds from the southern edge of the triangle across the river to Norfolk.

The fever was somehow in the air. Armstrong just didn't know what was carrying it. He'd soon be too consumed by the epidemic to figure it out.

CHAPTER NINE
HELP ON THE WAY

AT some point during severe epidemics, many of society's pillars crumble and a community can't sustain itself. Norfolk and Portsmouth had landed at that moment. The two cities could no longer provide the necessities of life to their own people: not food, not water, not medical care. There was no such thing as declaring a state of emergency. No federal aid. No Salvation Army. No Red Cross.

It had only been forty-three days since Trugien treated the first cases in Gosport, and the fever clamped its jaws around the necks of both cities. The *Herald* warned on August 13: "The provisions are becoming scarce, and it will not be long before some of the afflicted will be suffering from starvation." Some victims, like the Irishman Stapleton, were too dehydrated to battle the virus.

Schoolfield, head of the Sanitary Committee in Portsmouth, seemed to be turning the corner in his fight with the fever. But with him still hospitalized, the committee was not issuing daily reports from doctors. Norfolk physician R.W. Sylvester died, becoming the first of many doctors who would fall victim that summer. A *Petersburg Express* correspondent, who was a Portsmouth resident on the Sanitary Committee, wrote that twelve people had died in Portsmouth each of the past two days, including a local doctor. Samuel Barron, commandant of the Navy Yard, was on his deathbed. Barron had vowed that the Yard would remain open as long as it had men to swing hammers, but one thousand of the fifteen hundred workers had already left town.

Reliable news, if that's what the local papers were printing, became difficult to come by. The *Norfolk Bulletin* announced that all of its employees had left and it would cease publication. The *Portsmouth Transcript* stopped publishing, too. The owner of the *Herald* was reported to be dying.

Commerce was sketchy: Two Bank of Virginia directors fled, so the bank shut down. William Collins, founder of the critical Seaboard and Roanoke Railroad, came down with the fever, but his trains kept running. In Norfolk, the Cains Hotel closed. The post office relocated away from downtown, taking over the Norfolk Academy building. Abiding by the law became an honor system: Norfolk's chief of police sickened with the fever. Two of Portsmouth's three police officers died, and the third one had all the symptoms.

The *Petersburg Express* correspondent summed up the situation:

> "OUR TOWN authorities are doing all they can, but the scourge is so widespread that it is beyond their capacity. We have to take care of not only the sick, but of other members of their families. There is much suffering among the poor and the sick. We are greatly in want of breadstuffs, particularly of meal."[122]

On August 14, Norfolk residents heard the most dire news yet: Mayor Hunter Woodis had tried to ignore his symptoms, but even active, healthy people could not will themselves through the virus. While tending to the city's sick, Woodis collapsed in the street. He finally went home to get medical attention.

On the day Norfolk heard that Woodis had come down with

the fever, a group of businessmen met in Philadelphia to discuss the situation in Virginia. Philadelphia had no great historic connection to Norfolk or Portsmouth. It did not have the geographic link that Baltimore or Richmond did, being a quick steamer ride down the Chesapeake Bay or the James River to the two Virginia cities. Philadelphia was a northern city in favor of abolition; Norfolk was decidedly not. The men in the room did have one emotional connection to what was going on: They understood from the 1793 epidemic and more than a dozen others in Philadelphia the depth of torment that yellow fever could inflict upon a city. That morning, even though the Virginia cities had not written to ask for aid, the Philadelphia men rounded up six hundred dollars—the equivalent of twenty thousand five hundred dollars today[123]—and mailed it to the two cities with a letter[124]:

"PHILADELPHIA, AUGUST 15TH, 1855.

To the Mayor of the City of Norfolk:
Sir: Enclosed please find Drexal & Co.'s (Bankers) draft, No. 1910, for six hundred dollars. This sum is the result of a collection made since 9 o'clock this morning, among a few of the merchants of this city, who have instructed me to remit it to you, to be distributed among the "Howard Associations" of your City, Portsmouth, and Gosport in the ratio of their respective populations, to aid the Associations in their noble work of alleviating the distress upon the dreadful scourge now prevailing in your midst.
                              In haste, respectfully yours,
                    Thomas Webster Jr., No. 7, North Wharves"

That was just the beginning. The group formed a committee, which published an announcement in the Philadelphia papers the next day that they'd hold a public meeting on August 16 to adopt measures for "the Relief of the Poor of Norfolk, Portsmouth, and Gosport, Virginia, now suffering under the ravages of yellow fever."

At the meeting, they named block captains, fifty of them, each of whom would create their own committees with the goal of hitting every house, on every street, in the main part of the city. They would solicit aid daily. Thomas Webster Jr., a thirty-seven-year-old shipping agent, was named chairman.

The next day, Webster sent a letter and a four hundred dollar check to D.D. Fiske, Portsmouth's mayor, and another six hundred dollar check to Norfolk Howard Association President William Ferguson. On the 18th, he again sent six hundred dollars to Norfolk and four hundred dollars to Portsmouth. Webster also asked a series of pointed questions, aimed at finding out what else Philadelphia could do for the two ailing cities. The expectation of the day was that the representatives in the cities, either the mayor or the head of the relief organization, would reply and confirm each contribution that was made. Webster wanted to know:

What is the daily mortality? Based on population, is a 60 percent to 40 percent Norfolk-to-Portsmouth allocation appropriate? Are they in need of medicine? Are they in need of food? "Are you in want of doctors and nurses? I have sent three to Norfolk, and the next that offers shall be sent to Portsmouth."

Immediately upon the committee's formation, a Philadelphia doctor named William H. Freeman volunteered to go to Norfolk. Significantly, Freeman had spent a good bit of time in the West Indies and understood the seriousness of treating yellow fever patients. Webster wrote a letter of introduction for Freeman to take with him to Norfolk. Freeman would be joined by Doctor Louis Martin y de Castro, a native of Cuba who had studied medicine in Philadelphia. Webster dispatched a third man, W.W. Maul, who had volunteered to nurse the sick. To Ferguson, Webster asked:

"By telegraphic dispatch I see the deaths in Portsmouth are eight per day in a population reduced to 2,000. Is this really so? Information about the disease and population and wants of the respective places is very much wanted; as we are all deficient here as to exact data, and the papers are contradictory."

The responses from Portsmouth and Norfolk revealed the extent that the newspapers had either intentionally downplayed the epidemic, or if given the benefit of the doubt, had not known.

On August 22, instead of Portsmouth Mayor D.D. Fiske responding to one of Webster's letters, a Town Council member named James Holladay replied. In the first lengthy response to Webster, Holladay explained the obliteration of everything Portsmouth had been.

Holladay said the population—formerly ten thousand people—had shrunk by half, maybe even more. He had spoken with one of the most active doctors in town who estimated that three hundred to four hundred cases of the fever had occurred just in Portsmouth, and both men suspected that was a conservative figure. Nearly one out of ten who remained in town were sick.

"The disease is remorselessly seizing upon those who are left, without sparing age, sex, or color," Holladay wrote Webster. "The daily mortality is now double what it was a week ago. Yesterday, there were seventeen deaths ascertained, this morning up to ten o'clock, there had been ten."

Seventeen deaths "ascertained" meant that those had been officially reported and logged on the Register of Deaths, which revealed two other things: More people were dying every day in Portsmouth than anyone imagined, and even more whose deaths were not reported had perished. The virus had entered a self-propagating loop, reaching out and grabbing more and new victims daily. The large number of those infected had given the mosquitoes a greater chance of ingesting the virus when they fed, then turning around and infecting more people.

Portsmouth's flimsy support structure had collapsed, Holladay reported. At least four of the town's doctors were down with yellow fever, leaving the healthy ones overwhelmed. They couldn't get to every patient who needed them. The real problem was the lack of nurses. Families with any financial means had already fled, so the majority of residents were now from the under crust of society: those who couldn't afford a ticket on a steamer out of town, the enslaved, or freed Blacks who were not permitted to leave. Though doctors were all but certain that someone tending a sick family member could not contract the virus from them, regular people weren't so sure.

> "IN MANY CASES, there is not a soul to attend the sick and dying, but the undertakers, employees (his hearse driver, and driver's companion) to put the dead into their coffins and graves," Holladay wrote to Webster. "Literally the sick attend the sick, and almost literally, the dead bury their dead. In conclusion, sir, I will be frank with you. Our population is mainly a mechanical one and most of our people are dependent on daily labor for support. This disease has deranged every department of business, and is prevailing to a greater or less degree in almost every family."[125]

That same day, a man named Dulton Wheeler, secretary of the Norfolk Howard Association, also replied to Webster. Wheeler did not inform Webster that the mayor was down with the fever, but as with the Portsmouth reply, he peeled away the local papers' downplaying of the epidemic and laid out the unvarnished truth.

Wheeler estimated that more than two-thirds of Norfolk residents had fled, leaving behind about five thousand people in a city that had sixteen thousand residents just a month earlier. Norfolk had three hundred people struggling with the fever in their homes and another seventy at Julappi Hospital. The day before, the fever had sent fourteen Norfolk residents to the grave. Up until 10 a.m. on this day, there had already been eleven. If Philadelphia had any more doctors or nurses accustomed to treating yellow fever, Norfolk would put them to good use. One of the city's best physicians came down with the fever the day before, and he had been treating eighty victims. His cases would have to be spread among the other already overtaxed doctors. Wheeler added:

> SHOULD YOUR KIND letters not be promptly and satisfactorily answered, do not think hard of it, as we have so much to do and so few to do it.
> In regards to your kindness, what shall we say? Words are useless; but every one of our hearts are full of thankfulness and gratitude for our Philadelphia friends,
> In much haste, D. Wheeler, secretary

Within days of Philadelphia's first contribution, other cities, towns, and private citizens began writing letters and sending donations or making other offers to help. Fredericksburg, Virginia, residents met the day after Philadelphia at their courthouse and adopted a resolution. It informed Norfolk and Portsmouth citizens that Fredericksburg had a healthy atmosphere, did not have a quarantine against them, and welcomed refugees.

From Baltimore, James D. Mason & Co., a bread company, sent twelve barrels of wine biscuit.[126] A man in Franktown on Virginia's Eastern Shore wrote to Woodis offering Norfolk residents "the hospitalities of my house until the disease is allayed." A correspondent from Red Sulphur Springs, one of the springs resorts that the well-off had fled to, mailed one hundred dollars. He noted that fifty dollars of that had been contributed by President Franklin Pierce.

A Norfolk resident wrote Woodis saying that, if any of the people in Woodis's house should die and they didn't have a place to bury them, he would give up two plots that he owned in Elmwood Cemetery. A Baltimore company offered a supply of ice cream and "we would send it with or without flavor, as you might direct."

The residents of Savannah, Georgia, having been the recipients of aid from around the country the previous year during their epidemic, collected five hundred dollars. Two days later, Savannah sent another $1,272, the equivalent of more than forty-three thousand dollars today. A man named James French offered his residence near Old Point Comfort, as healthy a spot as can be found, he noted. The offer included two six-room cottages, a kitchen with four rooms, and use of the cistern water and outhouses. "Please use them as they were your own, free of all charge as long as you wish, either as a hospital or by residents," he wrote. "Mr. William B. Barnes, near Old Point, has the keys," French added. A man in Elizabeth City, North Carolina, volunteered a seventy-acre field at the edge of the confluence of the Chesapeake Bay and James River in case the Howard Association wanted to erect temporary buildings or tents and move residents from the infected cities.

A man named H.B. Sweeney wrote to Woodis. Little did he suppose, Sweeney wrote, that when he and Woodis attended college nearly two decades ago that they'd next connect during a catastrophe like this. Sweeney sent $258.50.

The funds and the help were critical to the survival of Norfolk and Portsmouth. The Howard Association paid the owner of a shuttered restaurant to reopen and serve soup to anyone who could get there. The association took over a warehouse owned by the Baltimore Steam Packet Company and converted it to a provision store.[127] Both moves created easy access to food and other supplies for family members tending to the sick.

The influx of help also added a significant load of work for the civic leaders who had stayed behind. More and more tasks fell to fewer and fewer people. In Portsmouth, just three people shouldered the load, as Winchester Watts wrote to his brother. The fever had struck Mayor D.D. Fiske and his family: "I shall be compelled for want of time to be brief. I have many letters to reply to. The carriage is waiting. I am going to the Naval Hospital to superintend the removal of the little destitute children to the Academy. I can get no one to go. Must perform the duty myself."

Watts and the Sisters of Charity dispatched to Portsmouth shepherded twenty-six orphans out of the hospital. The oldest were five or six years old. Some were just a few months old, not yet walking or talking, so the Sisters had the additional task of giving the children names.

Everywhere Watts went in town, every job he tended to, seemed to necessitate even more work. He had kept up his appearance by walking to a barber shop every day and shaving. One morning, he arrived to find the barbers trying to work while sick. He wrote notes for them and sent them all to the Naval Hospital.

He got a note that his brother's home insurance was expiring and had to deal with that. He visited his sick friends at the hospital. He kept his business, the icehouse, operational, because fever victims needed ice chips to alleviate their thirst. He attended funerals. He heard of a destitute family, visited their house, and found the mother scrambling for food and water for her sick child, with the father in the hospital. Watts wrote her an order to obtain provisions with relief funds. He was worn to the bone, yet he wouldn't let himself stop.

When the epidemic broke out, Portsmouth had eight practicing physicians, and now five had come down with the fever. One died. Watts wrote to the mayor of Baltimore asking if the city had any doctors who would volunteer to come down. Watts estimated Portsmouth's population had shrunk to about fifteen hundred to two thousand. "Considering the small number of us left, the mortality has been greater than it ever was in New Orleans," he wrote.

Watts occasionally lightened the mood of his reports with humor. One day, he told his brother as he signed off that he was about to head over to the Academy to check on the orphaned children. "The Sister of Charity who is in charge of them is very pretty . . . I think I shall fall in love with her."

The good news for the rest of the East Coast was that, even with refugees from Norfolk and Portsmouth finding clever ways to escape, the fever had not spread to other cities. They began to reopen their doors to residents who had remained behind. On August 18, Richmond citizens held a meeting to discuss how they could help.

Their first action was to invite Portsmouth and Norfolk residents to evacuate to Richmond and "its pure air, ample accommodations, and warm hospitalities." They resolved to ask the Richmond City Council to abolish the quarantine; those arriving in Richmond with yellow fever would be sent immediately to city hospitals or infirmaries. They'd also ask steamboat owners to resume regular trips up the James River from the two cities. If the city leaders didn't abolish the quarantine, they could land at the quarantine station on the river and transport passengers into the city from there.

A man then approached the chairman of the meeting with a letter from Thomas Dodamead, superintendent and agent of the steamer *Augusta*. Dodamead wrote that he would have attended in person, but he was sick and confined to his house. The owners of the *Augusta* contributed one hundred dollars toward provisions.

"I tender the use of the steamer *Augusta*, on behalf of the owners to transport provisions to their destination free of charge," Dodamead wrote.

A representative of the owners of the steamer *Curtis Peck* also offered free use of their ship to transport provisions or volunteers, and they arranged to legally haul refugees up to Richmond. They would rendezvous in the waters of Hampton Roads with the smaller steamer, the *Coffee*, whose passengers could transfer onto the *Curtis Peck* for the journey to Richmond.

At this point, this arrangement would help greatly with provisions but save few people. Enslaved people could not travel, and it was risky for freed Blacks even if they had the money—they could be mistaken for the enslaved and be jailed or sold. Most of the remaining Whites were either too sick to travel, or their family members were too sick. And folks like Woodis, Armstrong, and Watts had already made the call to bunker in and try to help the towns survive.

To them and everyone else, what time, what day of the week, what month it was, all became irrelevant. The only goal was to make it through the day, get some sleep, wake up, and redo the whole scene. One day at a time.

Watts's letters to his brother, Samuel, turned dire. "I felt quite sick this morning," he wrote on August 17, "and I thought I should have to go to the hospital." Watts asked himself the questions many now asked about normal aches and complaints. Was he tired because he was working hard, or was it fatigue from yellow fever? Did his back ache from helping victims onto the hospital cart or from the onset of the virus? Was he jittery because of the threat of getting the fever or agitated because it was already attacking his nervous system? It was mental torture.

He didn't go to the hospital and wrote again the next day, on August 18:

"About eighty new cases yesterday. I cannot give you a list of the deaths. I believe we shall all die. I have not received a letter from you in the last two days."

He followed up the next day:

"MOST OF OUR PHYSICIANS are either sick or broken down. Dr. Maupin sick at the Hospital. Mrs. Dr. Schoolfield very ill. Times are awful. Scarcely anybody here to consult with. Have had a hard time with it. I still keep my spirits up. My regards to all.

Yours sincerely, Winchester
Have not heard from you for the last three days."

After that, Samuel Watts stopped getting letters from his brother.

As with Watts and Woodis, the virus appeared to be getting nearer and nearer to Reverend George Armstrong. His nephew, a man in his early twenties, spent several days and nights tending to a friend believed to be afflicted with typhoid fever. Armstrong knew the friend lived in a part of town that had seen a mushrooming of cases in the previous ten days.

On a stormy Saturday, Armstrong got back to his house on Noe's Court after making his rounds and found his nephew, Edmund James, extremely sick. Edmund had violent pain in the back of his head, he told Armstrong. Armstrong could see Edmund's eyes glazed over, the edges of his swollen tongue chewed raw, with a dark coating down the middle. Armstrong checked his pulse. It was pounding.

Armstrong went to the Howard Association, got supplies, and secured an experienced nurse to come and tend to his nephew. It didn't help. Five days later, Edmund passed away. All of Edmund's friends who had tended the young man with typhoid soon came down with the fever also.

For Armstrong, his nephew was the first member of his church, First Presbyterian, to die from the fever. More worrisome, the fever had now leapt into yet another part of the city. And it had invaded Armstrong's own home.

The comforting concept of an "infected district" vanished. No part of town was immune. Yellow fever was no longer an Irish problem. The virus was not "mild and manageable." No one was safe.

On the third Saturday in August, a balmy tropical wind cut across the cities from the southwest. The air blew from inland and carried whatever bred in the marshes toward the densely populated streets. Steady blowing rain in the morning led to afternoon thunder and lightning. The squall dumped eight-tenths of an inch of rain. It was the first downpour in nearly three weeks.

In about ten days, hundreds of new broods of *Aedes aegypti* mosquitoes would swarm into the air

CHAPTER TEN
IN PURSUIT OF A CAUSE

TWO years earlier, the city of New Orleans drew most of the attention when yellow fever ran amok in the Mississippi Delta. But like a careening tornado that touches down, bounces up, then touches down again, the epidemic hopped around to communities dotting the Gulf Coast.

After many weeks of setting virus brush fires along the Louisiana and Alabama coast, the epidemic sparked to life in Mobile. That happened to be where a surgeon named Josiah Clark Nott lived with his wife and children. Nott's observations that summer would become central to the science of the day. His training at the New York College of Physicians and Surgeons, followed by the University of Pennsylvania Medical School, along with what he saw himself while living in Mobile, placed him firmly at the head of the pack of scientists and doctors trying to figure out how yellow fever spread. Nott's firsthand investigations into the movement of the virus that summer of 1853, along with previous publications of his observations in the 1840s, put him closer to the truth than anyone who came before him.

Nott certainly had his critics, stemming from his ongoing theorizing about Blacks. He contended that people from Africa originated from separate, inferior genetic makeup, which necessitated them being enslaved permanently.[128] Some Northerners wrote him off, deriding and dismissing his theories on that and everything else, while Southerners upheld his theories to burnish their support of a slave-based economy.

The spring of 1853, the outbreak started along the Gulf, as usual, with the arrival of a ship. With the New Orleans harbor taking in infected ship after infected ship, the debate was not whether a ship had brought yellow fever but which ship or ships had imported it. The barque *Siri*, a three-masted sailing ship, could have planted the seeds of the virus when it arrived from Rio de Janeiro on May 10. Rio had been a breeding ground for yellow fever since late 1849. The *Siri's* captain admitted upon arrival in New Orleans that he had lost his wife and two children to the fever in Rio.[129]

The ship *Home* docked on May 3. It lost many of its crew and the captain's wife on the way from Rio to Kingston, Jamaica. The captain recruited a new crew in Jamaica and set out for New Orleans. Or it could have been the *Northampton*, which in early May landed in New Orleans from Liverpool, England. Several of the four hundred passengers on the *Northampton* died crossing the Atlantic. Hands sent on board to clean the ship after it arrived in New Orleans discovered black vomit in the hospital ward.

Then there was the *Augusta*, which came in after a sixty-six-day passage from Bremen, Germany, via West Africa. The *Augusta* had been escorted into New Orleans alongside the *Camboden Castle*, a ship that had stopped in Kingston, a standard hotbed port. A sailor on the *Augusta* came down with the fever, remained on board while he battled the virus for fifteen days, and survived. The *Augusta's* cook then caught the virus and died.

Newspapers didn't report the outbreak for two months, after more than three hundred people had died. They sat on the news because Know Nothings ran the city, and the papers stayed loyal to the governing party. There was little concern as long as it only slayed the Irish, Germans, and other "non-Americans." The New Orleans

Daily Picayune ran a commentary that mocked "Madam Rumor" for the imaginary cases of yellow fever in the city, snarking that the "enormous" number of four cases had been reported. The editor of the *Daily Crescent* whistled past the graveyard, writing that yellow fever had become an "obsolete idea in New Orleans" and chastised city residents who had fled to what the paper called less healthy climates up north. The *Crescent* did mention "the buzzing and biting of mosquitoes," though even that had an upside: Cultured men who would not smoke in the presence of women could now use the mosquitoes as a reason to light up.[130]

Doctors hesitated to announce the cases, under the fear they'd be blamed for shutting down trade. Besides, they could not come to a collective diagnosis of what they were seeing. Doctor Erasmus Darwin Fenner, who treated numerous early cases at Charity Hospital, explained, "Some thought the subjects were too yellow, others that the yellowness was not the right hue . . . some said what was pronounced black vomit was not dark enough, others that it was too black. Some would not admit the cases were yellow fever, because they occurred too early in the season."[131]

By July, deaths piled up: two hundred one week, four hundred the next, nine hundred a week, twelve hundred a week. In the last week of August, in one seven-day period, 1,365 residents died of yellow fever.

It was in July that a ship named *Miltilades* sailed from Portland, Maine, to New Orleans harbor, where several crew died. *Miltilades* then set out for Mobile, Alabama, and anchored at a place called Dog River Bar. Nott and his family hunkered down that summer at his father-in-law's house in a nearby burg called Spring Hill, about ten miles from Mobile Bay. Nott had been worried for the city, as well as for his wife and seven children, as soon as he heard of the first deaths in New Orleans. Like everyone else, he had seen outbreaks emanating northward up the coast from Rio for the past four years. His father-in-law's house was not only inland from where cases usually struck first but also in a spot that hadn't been hit before.

The year after the 1853 epidemic, the New Orleans Sanitary Commission published its findings, along with written testimony of doctors, ships' captains, and others in a six-hundred-plus-page single-spaced report. The same would be done in 1855 by the sanitary committees and relief agencies of Norfolk, Portsmouth, and Philadelphia. The idea was to summarize the happenings, figure out how to prevent another epidemic, and advance scientific understanding. One of the physicians that the New Orleans commission reached out to was Nott. Buried among page after page of testimony is his submission, a lengthy and detailed response.

Nott first set about to slay miasma theory, the idea that Benjamin Rush, Noah Webster, and others propagated after the 1793 epidemic in Philadelphia. Though Rush had died four decades earlier and Webster ten years earlier, their bad-air hypothesis continued to muddle scientific advancement. Their publications and undercutting of other theories had been so effective that they still dominated cities' actions sixty years later. But the tactics they had used to discredit nearly every counter theory—that yellow fever was an American plague and only Americans could opine on it—would not have worked with Nott. He'd lived through epidemics in Mobile in 1837, 1839, 1842, 1843, and 1847.[132] In the midst of that, he spearheaded a group of doctors to form the Mobile Medical Society to take on the constant threat of yellow fever epidemics. The Alabama legislature sanctioned the group as a permanent Board of Health in 1842. Nott was as American as Irish hatred.

The only counter theory to miasma had long been the very incomplete argument that ships somehow imported the virus, but Nott did not set his sights on proving that. He began by conceding what everyone knew: "We are in the dark to the laws by which epidemic diseases are propagated." He knew full well the standing opinion: Decomposing animal or vegetable matter created foul-smelling gases, which then spread yellow fever. If true, Nott asked, how could this miasmatic gas infect a few houses on a street, skip several blocks, then start sickening people again? If spreading as a gas, how could the outbreak have hit Montgomery and Spring Hill—forty miles apart—at the same time? How was it, Nott asked, that the outbreak traveled up the Mississippi and around the Gulf Coast to only places where ships docked or trains stopped? A gas would not need a ship or train to move around.

"We can readily believe that certain insects . . . might attack only part of a ship," Nott wrote, "but we cannot imagine how a gas could be turned loose on one side of a cabin of a vessel and not extend to the other!!! Some new law of gases or emanations must be discovered by the Malaria party before they can explain this mystery."

Nott latched onto the concepts of an English geologist and biologist named Charles Darwin. Darwin had famously spent five years navigating the world on an English warship, the HMS *Beagle*, in the 1830s. On that trip, he found that existing scientific thinking could not explain how certain species had proliferated or wound up located where they were. Nott pointed out that Darwin had observed that insects and germs may lie dormant, then blossom to life when their "appropriate stimulus is applied."[133]

In one published paper, Nott explained that for long-time locals living on the Gulf of Mexico, swarms of insects were such an everyday event that it was a waste of breath to discuss them. At the moment he was writing, he said, he was so under siege by clusters of gnats, moths, and other bugs that people up north would find it inconceivable "how I can connect two sentences together. Facts that are before us constantly cease to excite reflection." The answer wasn't right under his nose; it was clamped onto his arm and drawing blood.

Nott, unlike nearly everyone else, was reflecting on insects. The theory that they were spreading the yellow fever germ, as he called it, made a hell of a lot more sense than anything else. Five years before the 1853 New Orleans and Mobile epidemic, Nott surmised that insects were best suited to the job. He mentioned moths, flying ants, aphids, and "the night mosquitoes."

"They remain quiet through the day, and do their work at night," Nott wrote. "We can well understand how insects wafted by the winds should haul up on the first tree, house or other object, but no one can imagine how a gas or emanation . . . could be caught in this way."

Nott wrote to the New Orleans Sanitary Commission that he considered his argument against miasma theory to be so settled that he was "not disposed" to debate it again. He didn't know how, but he'd seen yellow fever and other diseases "spring up from germs which have long been slumbering." But he couldn't prove his theories to anyone's satisfaction. The scientific method wouldn't come into play until the next century. Louis Pasteur's germ theory, which would eventually slam the door on Rush's miasma theory, would not take shape for another decade or more.

That summer and fall in Mobile, the fever decimated the city and surrounding villages, killing 1,191 people.[134] Nott wrote to the New Orleans Sanitary Commission that unlike in previous epidemics, that summer's outbreak spared no one. It struck down White people and Black people, long thought to have been immune; it struck Creoles, Irish, and Germans; it laid waste to people in old houses in swampy areas and people in new houses on high ground.

"Children who heretofore have been little liable, this year have been generally and violently attacked," Nott explained.

Nott knew that firsthand. Fever broke out in his family that summer. Four of Nott's seven children caught the virus and died.[135]

IN 2019, University of Washington researchers trapped two hundred fifty female *Aedes aegypti* mosquitoes in a container and pumped cold air inside to slow them down. Then they put the mosquitoes on ice to make them go to sleep. They then inserted them into a ten-by-fifteen-inch flight simulator, then tethered them to it with tiny wire pins and ultraviolet glue. When UV lights shined on the glue, it hardened to affix the pins to the mosquitoes. Inside the simulator, the animals turned into something akin to a wind sock—they could flap their wings and pivot but could not go anywhere.[136]

Researchers wanted to see what triggered their instincts to zero in on a person. They installed rows of light-emitting diodes to surround the mosquitoes, then used an infrared light to mark and time the shadows of beating wings. Then they blew in carbon dioxide, the gas that comes out of humans when they breathe. They projected an image that simulated a person against the side of the flight simulator.

Scientists found that the mere smell of carbon dioxide caused the *Aedes aegypti* to beat their wings furiously. When they projected an image of a person into the chamber, it caused the mosquitoes to beat their wings faster, but only slightly. But when the researchers stopped pumping the carbon dioxide, the mosquitoes barely showed an interest in finding the person.

"What their sense of smell is doing is telling them there's something there to investigate," Jeff Riffell, a University of Washington biology professor, told the *Seattle Times*. "Their vision tells them where the source of the smell is located."

Though yellow fever long ago disappeared from the United States, *Aedes aegypti* mosquitoes did not. Their presence is once again becoming relevant to Americans. Climate change has enabled the deadliest animal on Earth to expand its range in the United States. And it has managed to evolve. Of the three thousand five hundred species of mosquitoes in the world, only a few have adapted to live with and feed from humans. *Aedes aegypti*, the yellow fever mosquito, has morphed itself into one of the deadliest. It spreads yellow fever, dengue, Zika, and chikungunya, and sickens more than one hundred million people a year.[137]

Aedes aegypti now feed on humans to such a degree that scientists have genetically identified two related, but different, subspecies: the "wild" or forest-breeding one that still lives in Africa and the domestic one that developed its own feeding methods and shelter preferences after hitchhiking on slave ships to points all over the world. The human-targeting subspecies silently patrols the streets of places such as Saudi Arabia, Pakistan, Turkey, and Mexico. And get this: The deadly domestic *Aedes aegypti* lives comfortably in Florida, Georgia, Houston, Arizona, and among many other US locales, including Washington, DC. Each year that the winters become milder in the US, *Aedes aegypti* increases its presence.[138] These mosquitoes have been found in small populations as far north as New York and New England. As things stand, they circulate in locations where half the world's population resides.

Anywhere *Aedes aegypti* lives, it can become deadly the instant a new virus emerges. The World Health Organization, not known for melodramatic writing, detailed the mosquitoes' method of feeding on people as "sneak attacks." They avoid notice by striking victims from behind, then biting ankles or elbows. For people, it's tough to swat and kill something they don't see coming.

If a person does swat, scientists have discovered that mosquitoes have another self-preservation mechanism: Not only do they detect people with a keen nose for carbon dioxide, but they can differentiate among humans. Scientists have shown that mosquitoes can associate a specific smell with a certain act, such as swatting.

It took just fifteen minutes for a mosquito to associate a smell with a simulated swat. Not only that, but they also quickly began choosing hosts other than the swatter to land on, and they seemed to avoid the swatter's smell for the next twenty-four hours. "It means they can learn associations about who is more defensive and who isn't," Riffell said. "Their learning ability makes them incredibly flexible."[139]

When an *Aedes aegypti* mosquito lands on someone to feed, its sneaky, fine-tuned attack often ends before the person knows it happened. They have a pump-feeding system that helps them probe skin, siphon up the blood, then take off in seconds. Scientists figured out how this happens by using live X-ray videos to record mosquitoes feeding. Mosquitoes, unlike many other insects, have two pumps attached to their proboscis to draw blood. This gives them a "burst mode." During burst mode feeding, the mosquito activates both pumps to suck up a huge gulp of blood at once.[140]

The mosquito's burst mode draws as much as twenty-seven times the amount of blood of its normal sip. It's as if instead of taking five minutes to fill up a gas tank, it only took eleven seconds.

Once a mosquito's belly is full, it still must get away without causing a ruckus. Takeoff becomes more cumbersome because its blood meal doubles or triples its body weight. Once again, mosquitoes tackle this issue with a technique unique to aerodynamics. Most flying animals use their legs to spring into the air, then flap their wings—it works well, but makes a calamitous scene. Picture a dove taking flight.

A mosquito's takeoff is clandestine. It first fires up its wings, revving them three times faster than most insects, about six hundred flaps per second. Instead of pushing off with their legs, mosquitoes rotate their bodies so their wings can unfurl over a longer distance. They go airborne in about the same time it takes for a fruit fly to take off but without exerting any detectable pressure on a person's skin. "Instead of going fast, they take their time, but they accelerate the entire time," said Sophia Chang, who studied mosquitoes at the University of California, Berkeley.[141] "That is something that might be unique to mosquitoes, and maybe even unique to blood feeders."

Add to that *Aedes's* knack for hiding her eggs in plain sight. She'll drop a batch of a hundred or more eggs in a vase at a cemetery, another in a pet's water bowl, a bottle cap, even in the befouled water of a septic tank, or clogged gutters, or used tires. When they hatch, they'll find places to hide and will feed off a person when the opportunity arises. A female—males are simple creatures and only eat plant nectar—is willing to hide and wait for the right moment. She will duck under a bed, behind a dresser, in a shower stall, behind the washing machine or refrigerator. While they are aggressive daytime feeders, they've again learned from and adapted to human habits. At night, if they are in a house and a little light is left on, they'll bite then too.[142]

Aedes has all these techniques, tools, and tricks, and is prolific. In her short, three-week lifespan, an *Aedes aegypti* can lay at least three and as many as five batches, each with one hundred to two hundred eggs. It's easy to see the math that would lead to a mushrooming mosquito-fomented epidemic in a city or town with all the right conditions: People living close together, storms leaving behind standing water, streets or yards that don't drain well, and a virus circulating in more and more people—in other words, places like Norfolk and Portsmouth in the summer of 1855.

CHAPTER ELEVEN
The Fight to Exist

O N August 23, at 9 p.m., Doctor John Trugien arrived home. He'd been skittering around Portsmouth tending to the sick since 5 a.m. He'd seen and prescribed for one hundred patients during that sixteen-hour double shift, and he was frustrated about the patients he couldn't get to. He was treating not only his own patients but those of his mentor, Doctor Schoolfield, and another doctor, both of whom were down with the fever. Just three of Portsmouth's resident doctors were healthy and practicing. Trugien knew of victims whom no one had visited. He knew entire families who were sick and confined to their homes with no one well enough even to give them a drop of water. Added to that, every time Trugien stepped out of a sick person's house and headed for the next, people would come up to him and plead: Can you just spare a minute to tend to my father? Can you check on my mother? Would you please detour a bit to look at my brother?

Emotionally and physically, Trugien was wiped out. But he had one more task before he could sleep. Portsmouth streets were dark, and only a last gasp of sunlight tinted the summer sky. He would have had the windows open in his house to let in the cool night air. The flicker of a candle lit his spot. He grabbed a pen and paper and wrote to the editor of the *Petersburg Express*:

> "I AM NO ALARMIST, and have no disposition to exaggerate, but it would sicken anyone to know what is now transpiring in our town. I wrote to you yesterday a note designed for publication, beseeching medical aid. I know it must require an amount of courage possessed by few to venture thus seemingly into the jaws of death to rescue others. But is there no devoted man—no gallant soul—who will say I will go? Two or three physicians, I see, have volunteered for Norfolk, where the medical corps is larger than in this place. Shall poor stricken Portsmouth be left to her fate?"[143]

Trugien was right. The Philadelphia committee had sent two doctors to Norfolk—Louis Martin y de Castro and William Freeman. He didn't know that the committee had already vowed that the next doctors to volunteer would be allotted to Portsmouth. Nor could he imagine that his letter to the Petersburg paper would run in the larger *Richmond Dispatch* a few days later or from there that his passionate plea would reverberate up and down the East Coast. Though he felt isolated and unheard at the moment, his call for help worked. Soon, it seemed every time a steamer touched in the Virginia port, a doctor or nurse disembarked and reported for duty.

Three doctors took a steamer down the James River from Richmond and volunteer Henry Myers, a nurse, would join them in a few days after tending to half a dozen Norfolk residents who had fled to Richmond, then been hospitalized with the fever. Ten nurses departed from New Orleans two days after Trugien's letter; Virginia residents who had fled to New Orleans took up a collection to pay for the nurses' travel. Three Baltimore doctors took a steamer down the Chesapeake Bay and began tending to the sick the moment they arrived. They came, too, from Charleston, Savannah, Mobile,

Washington, DC, New York, and the West Indies, and one volunteer arrived from London.

As usual, Philadelphia stepped up in large fashion: Thomas Webster, chair of the Philadelphia Relief Committee formed just ten days earlier, wrote letters of introduction and dispatched four doctors and seven nurses to Norfolk. Trugien's call that Portsmouth had been forgotten hit home with Webster: He sent five doctors and five nurses to Portsmouth. Philadelphia not only sent money, doctors, and nurses, but Webster made sure its residents heard the specifics of what was needed and who was suffering.

Philadelphians locked in on the fact that Norfolk and Portsmouth were "mechanical towns," their economies stoked by hard labor rather than by medical, legal, and financial employment. People in the two cities made stuff: bricks, hats, wagons, barrels, ropes, boots, pumps, guns, and candy.[144] And they built ships. On August 26, workers at the Philadelphia Naval Shipyard banded together and donated $909.17. "This contribution," Webster explained to Portsmouth Mayor D.D. Fiske, "is made up of one day's pay of the master workmen, mechanics, and laborers employed at the navy yard." It was the equivalent of about thirty-one thousand dollars today. In a week and a half, Philadelphia had sent to Norfolk and Portsmouth nearly ten thousand dollars, equivalent to three hundred forty thousand dollars now.

The nurse volunteers may have been more important than the doctors or the money. It is known now and was beginning to come to light then that the only effective treatment for a yellow fever victim is supportive care. If patients had nurses who could keep them comfortable and hydrated, they stood a decent chance of living.

But fear and rumor dictated behavior. People were so terrified of getting the fever that many would not even enter the bedroom of sick family and friends. Those who braved entering a sick person's room covered their faces with bags of camphor or asafoetida, odoriferous herbs imported from Asia. Even then, they were afraid to get near enough to hand their sick relative or friend a glass of water.

"You may tell them as often as you choose that the disease is not contagious; they will not believe you, and it is useless to talk to them," a *Dispatch* correspondent wrote. "On this account nurses are difficult to obtain, and many perish merely for the want of attention."

The nursing of Annie Andrews and the Sisters of Charity was making a difference over at the old racetrack along the Elizabeth River. Those running the Norfolk relief effort sent what seemed like the most hopeless cases to the hospital. They fitted up a barge, spreading mattresses for the sick across much of the deck and erecting supports for an awning to protect the sufferers from the Southern sun. People called it the "Plague Boat." A man who docked near it one day documented what he saw on board: two men, one a father who most assuredly would die, three boys about eight to ten years old, a little girl about four years old, and a coffin. The father's hat kept falling off as he slumped over, and the girl would gently place it back on top of his head.

With about seventy patients at Julappi Hospital, Andrews and the three Sisters of Charity hustled from bed to bed all hours of day and evening. They took shifts sleeping. The *Dispatch* reporter paid a visit to Julappi. What he saw impressed him. "The true place for those sick with the fever is the Hospital at Lambert's Point," he wrote. "There is pure air, no infection, prompt treatment and kind nursing." He reported that in the past twenty-four hours, only two patients at the hospital had died.

Despite the help, with hundreds of people sick in both cities, the nursing shortage would persist throughout the epidemic. The White residents expected that the Black people living among them would step forward since the perception lingered that those of African origin were biologically immune to yellow fever. When Black people refused to step into, as Trugien put it, the "jaws of death," the rest of the community couldn't understand why. "The greatest difficulty was experienced in procuring nurses," the *Dispatch* reported, "the negroes refusing to act in that capacity at $10 a night. $5 a night had previously been paid for the service."

In 1855 Virginia, Black people were only included in the conversation when their work was in demand. All other times, they didn't count. Whites would talk about how many people had fled Portsmouth: *Only fifteen hundred out of a White population of eight thousand remained.* Or how many people they saw: *I walked four blocks and did not see any other White people.* But they were a significant part of life in the cities. In Norfolk, for instance, the 1850 Census showed the city had a population of 14,320, which included 4,295 enslaved people and another 957 free Blacks. The number of free Blacks had declined over the previous decade "due to the view now generally known by Southern men to be correct, that freedom is not beneficial to the African when it is in contact with the white race."[145] The city's number of enslaved Africans jumped 15 percent during the decade.

The idea that Black people were born immune to yellow fever emerged from legitimate observations. In early epidemics, fewer people of African origin had sickened and died from the virus than Whites. Some had seemed downright impervious. The truth, of course, is that they'd probably been immunized the hard way—by contracting the virus and surviving it, when no one paid much attention. Those who could be proven to be acclimated fetched a higher price. The hitch in 1855 was this: Enslaved Africans had been hauled into Southeast Virginia since the early 1600s. Many of the Black people in Norfolk and Portsmouth had been born there. They had just the same probability as the White people to have become immune during a previous epidemic—a slim chance, since the last major epidemic had been in 1826.

The thinking that Black people were immune may not have started in Philadelphia, but like many lessons learned from the 1793 epidemic, the concept solidified then and hopscotched to other coastal cities. Once again, the famous signer of the Declaration of Independence, America's name-brand doctor, Benjamin Rush, helped write that narrative.

Rush strongly advocated for the abolition of slavery, and among his missions in Philadelphia was to be a catalyst for more conversation and collaboration among Whites and Blacks. Pennsylvania had officially outlawed slavery in 1780, and by 1800, only a few dozen enslaved Africans lived in the city and as many as six thousand free Blacks. Of course, multiple forms of almost-slavery existed, like domestic servants, indentured servitude, and abysmally low pay for back-breaking work.

Rush befriended two influential free Black men in Philadelphia, Richard Allen and Absolom Jones, who had founded the Free African Society, an organization that provided financial support to Black people for health care and burials. Jones had been born into slavery in Delaware; his mother, sister, and five brothers were sold, and Jones's enslaver brought him to Philadelphia, where he was freed. He learned to read and write well by studying the Bible. He teamed up with Allen to form First African Church, and they petitioned the Episcopal Diocese of Pennsylvania to join.[146] The Diocese brought the church into its fold, and it was renamed African Episcopal Church. Rush helped found it.

When yellow fever began sickening and killing Philadelphians by the hundreds in 1793, the mayor, with Rush as a conduit, approached Jones and Allen for help. The belief by many that Black people were immune to yellow fever may have been born of observation, but it was also eminently convenient. If Black people were immune, they would not be risking their lives to venture into the sickest parts of town to nurse White people. Jones and Allen, hopeful that their church members and other Black people would become accepted members of society, agreed to help convince their flock to volunteer as nurses. And they did, hundreds of them. And they died, hundreds of them.

For seventy days that summer and fall, the Black nurses not only tended the sick, they lifted the ailing into carriages to send them to hospitals when the victims' own family members would not; they cared for the victims' children; they even bought coffins with their own money. They got little thanks for any of it. Matthew Carey, an Irish immigrant, became the top chronicler of the Philadelphia epidemic due to his prolific writing. His book, *A Short Account of the Malignant Fever Lately Prevalent in Philadelphia*, became the Bible of the epidemic. In the book, Carey conceded that the fever did hit the Black population, though he said the number was "not great." He wrote that many of the volunteer Black nurses "demand public gratitude," but alleged that they took advantage of ailing White people by "plundering the houses of the sick." He said they were price gouging the sick, charging as high as five pounds a night.

Carey's words stung. Jones and Allen, unlike almost all other members of their race, had the standing and wherewithal to correct the record. The two struck back with eviscerating precision. They published their own account, *Proceedings of the Black People During the Late Awful Calamity in Philadelphia and Refutation of Censures*.

They first pointed out that, while they stayed in Philadelphia to tend to the dying and the dead, Carey fled. "We feel ourselves sensibly aggrieved by the censorious epithets of many, who did not render the least assistance in the time of necessity yet are liberal of the censure of us."

After that head slap, they laid out a for-the-record account of how they became enlisted in nursing the sick, who they helped, and the price they paid, both in money and with their lives. They said they first responded to a solicitation in city newspapers for Black people to come forward to help the sick who couldn't get care, "with a kind of assurance that people of our colour were not liable to take the infection."[147] On the first day when a handful of Black volunteers came forward, they helped twenty families. They walked into situations, like a husband sick in the house with no one tending to him and his wife dying in the alley outside.

They worked with the mayor of Philadelphia; they worked with Rush and his medical faculty. After the sickness spread widely across the city "that good man Doctor Rush called us more immediately to attend upon the sick." Rush taught the Black nurses his bleeding techniques and his dosages for the calomel so his innovative techniques could reach more people.[148]

During the operation, Allen, Jones, and several others built an entire organization. They kept a ledger, retained receipts, and logged the visits, deaths, and burials. They paid more than three hundred pounds to hire five men to help hoist the dead onto carts, to carry others to the hospital, and to move the sick from room to room. They were never paid back for that, and often, they were too busy to care for sick members of their own families or their church. Jones estimated that more than three hundred Black people died that summer.

"When people of colour had the sickness and died, we were imposed upon and told it was not with the prevailing sickness, until it became too notorious to be denied," the men wrote. "Then we were told some few died but not many, thus were our services extorted at the peril of our lives, yet you accuse us of extorting a little money from you."[149]

They suffered equally with White people, yet few of the White population paid attention, even while being nursed by Black people. But the message landed a few years later when another epidemic struck Philadelphia. Despite the public begging for nursing help from the Black community, this time Black people stayed home and took care of their own.

Back in Norfolk, half a century later, Black people could not be convinced to nurse the sick "for love or money." An enslaved man named John Jones did perform daily, heroic work. At all hours of early morning, the hot midday sun, right up until dusk put the day to bed, Jones steered a horse and carriage up and down Norfolk's streets to look for coffins to cart to the cemetery. Often, just Jones and one surviving family member would muscle the casket from the curbside up onto his wagon. Many times, the survivor would not even tag along to Elmwood Cemetery to unload and bury their loved one. Jones and whoever else was there to drop off another body would do that.

Jones's horse and wagon caught the eye and ear of the only people out and about, the ministers, doctors, nurses, and newspaper correspondents, along with the few residents well enough to go out for supplies. The Death Car, as they called Jones's carriage, turned heads as it clattered over cobblestones and rattled across potholes. At the front sat Jones, puffing continuously on a nine-inch cigar to keep away whatever was in the air. The White residents had talked it over: After the epidemic, they'd see about buying Jones his freedom, if he somehow survived.

At least this time around, people could no longer deny that the yellow fever virus attacked the Black population as well as the White. Doctor George Upshur, along with two colleagues, had years ago established a "slave infirmary" in Norfolk, and that hospital was maxed out. The Howard Association took over a building in town and fitted it up as a hospital for "the colored sick," the *Dispatch* reported. "So many of that class are attacked that such a step has become necessary."[150]

NORFOLK AND PORTSMOUTH had been clamped down in fear for more than a month. As the residents tried to just make it through August any way they could, anger heated up and rolled toward a boil. The owners of the steamer *Coffee*, which plied the waters of Hampton Roads from Portsmouth and Norfolk, over to Hampton, and out to Old Point, were ticked off at the commandant at Old Point Comfort for repelling boats that originated from Norfolk. Sentries guarded the docks and enforced the dictum with bayonets. The *Coffee's* owners announced they would sue the commandant for ten thousand dollars in damages.

Though Richmond and Petersburg had dropped their quarantines against residents of the Virginia port cities, animosity toward them hung in the air. A *Southern Argus* correspondent wrote that "under no circumstances should the Howard Association consent to receive one dollar from Richmond and Petersburg." Plenty of relief funds would come from Baltimore, Philadelphia, and New York, so the relief groups should send back contributions from Richmond and Petersburg's "narrow-hearted and unchristian Virginians." A new *Dispatch* correspondent, in reporting this, wryly noted that the writer datelined his letter from Hampton, a city devoid of starvation and sickness.

Into this sick and seething environment stepped a new correspondent for the *Richmond Dispatch*, a man who signed his posts with the outwardly righteous pen name VERDAD, Spanish for "Truth." He wrote long reports, yet he had a knack for stringing together powerful words that cut straight to the point. He lived in the middle of Norfolk, and he got out and talked to people. His first bulletin on August 22 noted twenty-two deaths up until 2 p.m. that day, "but there are altogether, including those who have been buried at Potter's Field, thirty."

He was poetic; he was melodramatic: "Truth compels us to say, from private observation, that no part of Norfolk is now free from infection, and that danger lurks everywhere within its borders."

VERDAD's honest assessment of the city's condition may come as sad news to friends and family in other cities or states, he admitted, but "as faithful chroniclers we intend to narrate the truth, nothing more, nothing less." Portsmouth and Norfolk had, in fact, developed new morality codes over the past six or eight weeks. They'd had to exist on their own for weeks, locked in by wide rivers, the only routes sealed shut by idled steamers and quarantine regulations. Money, land, property? They mattered much less now. What mattered was family, you, and whether you'd live. And what else mattered was loyalty. Had you stayed to help and done all you could? Or had you fled in your family and city's greatest time of need?

In his daily reports, VERDAD quickly sketched this new morality.

To him, there were no shades of gray, just heroes and villains. In his first article, he absolved Richmond for initially enacting a quarantine against the two cities; he figured it was done out of panic, much like what spurred Norfolk's own residents to a "hasty and early stampede. Under these circumstances, what more could we expect from strangers when our own people deserted their homes?"[151]

VERDAD raised high Mayor Hunter Woodis who "exposed himself in the faithful discharge of his duty" along with making honorable mention of Doctor Upshur and several others. He lauded Doctor Thomas Constable for hearing about the outbreak during a summer vacation at a springs resort and returning to Norfolk to tend to the sick. VERDAD listed by name two doctors who had been in town at the outset and fled to the springs to get away.

Then he moved on to the clergy, and it got nasty. He praised George Armstrong, William Jackson of Saint Paul's Episcopal Church, Lewis Walke of Christ Church, several others, and Father Matthew O'Keefe of Saint Patrick's Catholic Church as being "on the lips of everyone" for their dedication. VERDAD wrote that Protestants and Catholics together should "join together in paying deserved tribute" to those ministers. It was all just setting the table for VERDAD's righteous roast:

"The Minister of the Free Mason street Baptist Church is the only one who has proved recreant to his duty, and unfaithful to his flock. He left the city shortly before the epidemic broke out, and has kept himself safe away ever since. As a Christian minister he should have returned immediately . . . but in place, he wrote to know whether it would be safe for him to return."

With that, VERDAD transitioned to the grim duty of people who were sick or had died in the last forty-eight hours: Mister Greenwood, Reid's Lane; George Lee, Queen Street; son of W. Barnes, James Street; W. Steele, Bute Street; colored boy of E.T. Summers; Negro man Jack owned by Missus Good; Negro man at Doctor Cooke's; Negro man at John Gibbs's; Mister Dumott, an English gardener, found in a dying state in some bundles of fodder in an outhouse on Bute Street . . .

Then VERDAD wrapped up his first submission to the *Dispatch*, a thirteen-hundred-plus-word piece, with a fatalistic pledge:

"I WILL KEEP you advised of our unhappy state of affairs from day to day, as long as I am able to keep up.

VERDAD."

Along the way, he had tucked in a critical observation, hidden between his rant and the death report: The weather was hot, sultry, and showery. Many expected it to increase the number of new cases.

CHAPTER TWELVE
BEWILDERED

JOHN Trugien, the young Portsmouth doctor, sent his letter to the *Petersburg Express* pleading for medical help just in time. The day he dropped it in the mail, he came down with yellow fever. It was inevitable: Trugien's work had led him from the site of the first cases, yards from where the *Benjamin Franklin* docked, into the swampy, narrow streets of Gosport, and in fact had lured him from one outbreak hotspot to the next for the past two months. The result was no different than if he had volunteered for a medical experiment that required him to be bitten by *Aedes aegypti* mosquitoes.

VERDAD reported the news first, in an August 25 post:

"THE FEVER IN Portsmouth continues with unabated ravages. 500 cases under treatment. Many of the physicians are sick. Dr. Trugien is said to be very ill, and not expected to live."

The Naval Hospital admitted Trugien the same day his mentor, Schoolfield, was well enough to be discharged. Two days later, the papers reported that Trugien was doing well. The next day, the hospital staff summoned Schoolfield at 2 a.m. to say his farewells. Trugien's brain had already entered a state of delirium, and Schoolfield was certain his protégé did not recognize him. Trugien died hours later. Schoolfield penned a note to the *Petersburg Express*. After Trugien made his plea for help the previous night, he didn't sleep. Instead, he learned of a close friend who was sick and sat up all night with him. The next day, the fever engulfed Trugien.

> "THE SAD TASK devolves upon me of announcing the death of our dear friend, Dr. J.W.H. Trugien. 'He worked at the oar until he fell,' to use his words. Truly has fallen a good man. At some other occasion, I may express my views of his character, which deserves much more than a newspaper epitaph . . . I have not the heart to say more."

As was now the necessary custom, Trugien was buried the same day he died. Friends and admirers joined with visiting doctors from Charleston, Richmond, and Baltimore to pay their respects to Trugien and the dedication he had shown to his hometown. Tears rolled down the gravedigger's cheeks.[152]

It had been sixty days since Trugien treated the first cases in Gosport, and the fever barged into more homes, emptied the houses on more blocks, infected more people's blood every day. Those clinging to any whiff of optimism pointed out that deaths in Norfolk may have leveled off the past two days, with about thirty people a day being buried. In fact, no one really knew the number. VERDAD tossed cold water on that theory, correctly pointing out that new cases were "the great thermometer of the disease" and those were skyrocketing. Unlike any previous yellow fever epidemic in Norfolk, the virus oozed away from the harbor and breached north of what locals had long considered safe boundaries. VERDAD observed that as the virus began infecting a new part of town, families loaded wagons, carts, drays, whatever could haul their belongings, and fled toward the countryside "like chaff before a tornado."

Entire city blocks were now abandoned. The best anyone could estimate, approximately two-thirds of Norfolk's population had fled. Out of an original sixteen thousand people, about five thousand were still in town. Armstrong estimated that among that population, twelve hundred to fifteen hundred were sick. For every three people bitten by an *Aedes aegypti* mosquito, one would transmit the virus to the insect. Around and around the virus went.

"The pestilence, long darkling over us, has now burst upon us in its terrible might," Armstrong wrote.

Armstrong had never criticized those who fled the cities when the virus first leapt the river to Norfolk, but he had hoped more would stay. It would have tamped down the panic, he thought. Residents could have battled the virus as a united front. Now, six weeks after his friend Doctor George Upshur reported the first Norfolk cases, Armstrong had changed his mind. If everyone had stayed and sickened at the same rate, other East Coast cities could not have provided enough doctors and nurses, or enough food and medical supplies, for the sick. The city would have been crushed by its own weight. Even with all those who fled, he realized many were dying simply due to lack of care. He now viewed the residents' flight as "God's means of scattering them so they might be saved."

Collectively, the city donned a surreal cloak. Powdered lime swirled and clumped in standing water. Abandoned dogs roamed the streets in packs searching for food. Stacks of coffins stood on street corners, waiting for John Jones to clatter up in his "Death Car" carriage to haul them away. The cities' residents hadn't expected devastation at this level, the destruction of all normality, the disappearance or death of nearly everyone they knew and relied on. They were in shock.

"You have no doubt seen persons when some great calamity has come upon them—although all is not lost if they will exert themselves—sitting down in a sort of sullen indifference, bewilderment," Armstrong wrote on September 1. "Our people seem to be bewildered."

Mayor Hunter Woodis had died only a week earlier, and the

dazed residents already missed his leadership. Like Armstrong, Trugien, Schoolfield, the Catholic Priest Francis Devlin, VERDAD, and others, Woodis had spurned the thought of personal danger. He had been the one scurrying around the city to help victims, setting up the barricades to try to hem the virus into Barry's Row, organized the first relief from Philadelphia, and generally seemed to be tireless and bulletproof until the end. With Woodis's death, the most senior member of the City Council took his place. Armstrong knew N.C. Whitehead would do his best, but Whitehead also was president of Farmers' Bank, which he was trying desperately to keep open. "He is not the young, active man that Woodis was," Armstrong noted.

Amid this desperation, a bold idea began to circulate. VERDAD mentioned it first: The poor didn't have the funds for a steamer ticket out of town much less lodging to wherever they would flee, so why not find a way to help everyone who was well enough get out of town? "If a boat could be sent here to take away gratis those who are without means to escape, a large number of worthy but humble lives would be saved," the crusading journalist wrote. He wasn't the only one suggesting, essentially, to move the cities' populations.

Two days later, Philadelphia Relief Committee Chairman Thomas Webster wrote to Portsmouth Mayor D.D. Fiske and the Norfolk Howard Association. Webster explained that he had not previously had time to research suggestions for the cities, but he had now devoted some time to gathering recommendations. He had consulted with his friend Charles D. Meigs, from the Jefferson Medical College in Philadelphia. Meigs said that removing the populations from the infected districts, which now covered the entirety of both cities, was the most surefire way to save lives. He suggested petitioning the federal government immediately for tents and pitching them in an open, airy field. Fiske didn't respond, and Webster came back to the idea just days later.

"Why don't you remove your healthy population, and starve the fever?" Webster asked. "Pardon the freedom of my remarks, but after all, removal from infection is the surest plan of subjugating the fever."

Webster had scoured the Western Hemisphere for advice on caring for yellow fever patients. From a doctor in Pernambuco, a port city in northeast Brazil, Webster heard that mustard poultices applied to the abdomen, feet, and legs helped, along with ice held to the forehead. The absolute best treatment, the Brazilian doctor said, was pulverized ice—just the ice itself, not ice and water.

Webster got word that the US government had provided circulars detailing the meteorology, proximity to rivers, elevation, drainage, and position related to marshes to the New Orleans Sanitary Committee for its report on the 1853 epidemic there. Webster wrote to Secretary of State William L. Marcy and asked that copies of the circulars be mailed to the heads of the Norfolk and Portsmouth relief groups. Marcy found the last two copies and shipped them out.

Webster took it upon himself to become almost the personal concierge to the two relief associations. He tracked down any items they wanted. He suggested items they might need. He was frustrated, determined, thoughtful, and absolutely driven. "Should you not have liberal quantities of Bay Rum, Cologne water, aromatic vinegar, and likewise an abundance of lemons, arrow root, tapioca, sago, bare barley and oatmeal for the convalescent, let us know," Webster wrote.[153]

He suggested that the cities would surely need quinine, which along with calomel was the primary medicine used to treat yellow fever. The substances were so well-known that often people were administered adulterated medications. Philadelphia, Webster wrote, had one of the top quinine manufacturers in the world and perhaps the Virginia cities could benefit from a reliable supply direct from the factory. "What say you?" he asked.

Along the way, Webster found himself forced to weigh the morality of how Philadelphia helped. Usually, he had to make the determination by himself. Toward the end of August, he twisted himself into knots over one particular volunteer, a young woman named Leonora Patterson. The eighteen-year-old had recently converted to Catholicism and applied to be sent to Portsmouth as a nurse. Webster didn't feel right about sending such a young woman into, as Trugien had written, "seemingly the jaws of death." He'd been hesitant when a fifty-five-year-old widow had insisted on going but said yes. A teen-aged woman was too much.

"I positively refused, but may yet have to write her a letter," Webster wrote to Portsmouth's mayor. "The five 'Sisters of Mercy' have not yet left. Miss Patterson is not a sister, but was to go with them. If you can send back the Ice Cream cans and tubs, I need not pay for them. Deem it not parsimonious to call your attention to these items, for their value can be realized by your community in cash."

Webster tended to every wish, to needs that the Virginia cities had before they knew they had them. He tracked contributions, and if the Philadelphia group had not received a corresponding letter confirming the receipt, he followed up to confirm. He wrote letters of introduction for every doctor, nurse, and pharmacist the committee dispatched to Virginia, but he really didn't want to send the young Miss Patterson into the calamity. As part of his attempt to keep her in Philadelphia, he wrote to three prominent Catholic priests for help:

"FATHERS SHERIDAN, MCNANNY & MCGOVERN:

A Miss Leonora Patterson, aged eighteen, a recent convert to your church, persists in offering her services to go to Portsmouth as a nurse for yellow fever. She claims she has a right to go, because she intends devoting her life to religion and charity. Will you have the kindness to let me know something relating to her? I thought you might be cognizant of some information which would induce you to remonstrate with her against going."

Right after that, Webster wrote to Portsmouth Mayor D.D. Fiske, explaining the background then asking for Fiske to be the one to deny her request: "I have deferred giving her a letter under the hope that you will say positively that you are not in want of any more nurses."

Webster gave it his all, and he also knew it was a futile effort. The teenager would either go with the committee's introduction, or she'd go on her own. After all but begging Fiske to reject her application, Webster asked Fiske to personally watch over her: "My dear Sir, take her by the hand and let her go to the chambers of the sick and fill the sphere to which she devotes herself. Watch over her, too." Webster feared that, in the end, Patterson would need medical help from the relief committee herself.

A frightening quiet enveloped the parts of the cities that the fever had terrorized early on. Before the epidemic, the hardworking waterfront soundtrack set the pace of hourly life. The stevedores chanted sea songs as they loaded and unloaded ships, steady and methodical rhythms that matched the pace of the heavy lifting. The carpenters' hammers pounding on ships overlaid a faster, more frantic track. Machinery clanked and screeched in flourishes. Now, it was all gone.

The *Southern Argus* reported the change under the headline "Death's Quiet":

> "YESTERDAY, the slow and regular strokes of the old clock far up Freemason Street were distinctly heard at our office, not far from the river. The measured note sounded strangely and sadly, and fell upon the ear like the melancholy toll of a funeral knell."

The *Argus* was lucky to still be publishing. The *Portsmouth Transcript*, Mayor D.D. Fiske's paper, announced it was shutting down. The mayor had been forced to write the last issue, then set the metal type, work the press to print, and gather the copies to distribute them himself. It was too much for one man.

Norfolk's chief of police, Elias Guy, and his entire family were down with the fever. Reports of his illness, along with that of another one of his officers, left the city open to an every-man-for-himself mentality. William Forrest, the reporter and historian, was out sick with the fever. Captain George Chambers, superintendent of the ferry across the Elizabeth River between the two cities, died. And the fever infiltrated the home of Mayor Fiske, sickening him and his entire family. Even Annie Andrews, the first nurse volunteer, was reported to be sick. On both sides of the river, at least eight doctors were either sick or dead. VERDAD lionized the heroes and savaged the villains. As with all epidemics, there were plenty of both.

On August 26, VERDAD reported that the US Customs Office in Norfolk had moved itself across the water to Hampton, forcing the few still trying to import or export goods to travel. Such abandonment of a customs location had never occurred in previous yellow fever epidemics in the South, he wrote.

"If our custom house officers were afraid to remain at their post and do their duty like men, why did they not resign and leave their places to be supplied by others, fully as competent and with less pusillanimity, who would gladly have taken their fat berths?"

If the customs office could be moved, next might come the post office, and the Navy itself, VERDAD suggested. If so, why not move the city itself to Old Point and its "salubrious breezes of that airy locality."

There's no record the customs officers issued a response, but Reverend Tiberius Gracchus Jones of the Freemason Street Baptist Church issued a long retort of VERDAD's public shaming of him for fleeing town at the beginning of the outbreak. He wrote to the *Richmond Dispatch* and the editor of the *Norfolk Argus*. He lashed out a nearly two-thousand-word rebuttal—or an attempt at one. His first move was to strip VERDAD of his anonymity, naming R.T. Halstead as the writer, so it may be "known in Norfolk who it is that sought to disparage me."

Jones then took aim at the idea that heroes or villains existed amid the pestilence. Newspaper editors praised those who stayed behind or those who surged in to help, Jones said, assigning "saint" or "hero" labels while "ignorant of the true motives and circumstances which induced them to do so." He suggested that their "moral character" was not taken into account. Jones, in a public relations mistake, then requoted large sections of VERDAD's shellacking of his character. For readers who had missed the controversy the first time, Jones republished it for all to see. Then he did a poor job of defending himself and came across as a man who doth protest too much.

Before he left Norfolk, no members of the Freemason Street Baptist Church had caught the fever, and the poor who were dependent on the church had been taken care of, Jones argued. Before he could return, most of the congregation had left town. Those remaining would not likely attend church during an epidemic, he said.

"As for funerals, in such times, if I mistake not, they are not attended for want of ministers, except for those who suppose that prayers over the bodies of the dead benefit their departed souls," wrote Jones, seeming to question the very foundation of religious beliefs.

After all that, Jones wrote that he wasn't concerned that VERDAD's publicity would ruin his reputation. Everyone who knew the "peculiar circumstances" that forced him to vacate his post either advised him to leave or would understand why. However, those were "circumstances which I feel under no necessity of mentioning."

Jones's response left VERDAD unconvinced and undeterred. He wrote that he had not read Jones's letter himself, but friends who are good judges of such things told him not to bother, that Jones's response did not satisfy the public. "Nothing we could say could do Mr. Jones more harm than he has done himself." Then he reported on Jones's temporary stand-in:

"Rev. T.G. Keen arrived here yesterday to take charge for the present of the Freemason Street Baptist Church," he reported, "in place of the regular pastor who can't venture among us for a while."

While VERDAD was orchestrating his one-man morality symphony, he noted that yellow fever had broken out in the city jail. It had already killed one prisoner and sickened several others. "It would be an act of retributive justice if Goslin, imprisoned there awaiting his trial for the murder of Murphy, could fall victim to it. The principal witnesses against him have died, and he stands a fair chance of escaping should he survive the epidemic."

Armstrong got involved in the fracas over the Freemason Street Baptist Church after he picked up his mail one morning at the post office, which had been relocated out of downtown to the Norfolk Academy school building. The new post office grounds quickly became the place to meet up with whoever was still well enough to get there. That morning, Armstrong got a letter from a physician friend in Philadelphia. The doctor asked Armstrong about rumors that nearly all the Protestant clergy in Norfolk had abandoned their posts. Armstrong wrote back, telling his friend that he'd been so occupied visiting the sick and helping bury the dead that he had no idea such a report was circulating.

Armstrong detailed for his friend the whereabouts of the pastors of the eight White churches and two Black churches in the city. He conceded that both Baptist ministers had left town, one by prior arrangement, and that the pastor of Christ Church had gone to Germany before the crisis began. With seven out of ten at their posts, during summer when many would be traveling, Armstrong figured Norfolk's pulpits were as well staffed as in any city. He then left his friend with an ominous warning:

> "UNLESS A MIRACLE preserve us, there will be more than one green mound in our cemetery to bear witness to the falsehood of this report."

In fact, Armstrong had just returned from the funeral of Reverend Anthony Dibrell, pastor of the Granby Street Methodist Church. Dibrell had "fallen at his post," succumbing to the fever while at church among his parishioners. He was a popular minister, known all over the city by Methodists and non-Methodists alike. The paltry attendance at this funeral dismayed Armstrong; so few turned out it was hardly worth going through the traditional burial rites.

"His own son and I helped put his coffin in the hearse," Armstrong wrote.

Armstrong now had even bigger things to worry about. His twelve-year-old daughter had just recovered from what he said was a slight attack of bilious fever. This was a catch-all diagnosis, simply meaning she was vomiting a lot of bile. Often, bilious fever sufferers also took on a jaundiced appearance. She was prescribed a purgative and calomel, and Armstrong had hoped the recent infection and cleansing of her system would buffet her against other viruses.

"Instead of this, it seems to have laid the system more fully open to attack," he wrote.

Mary was now down with the yellow fever. Armstrong assessed that her case was a "mild and manageable one" and was hopeful she'd recover quickly.

On the last day of August 1855, something good finally happened in Portsmouth. On that day, one of the yellow fever patients at the US Naval Hospital beckoned for a pen and paper. For the first time in eleven days, Winchester Watts was well enough to write to his brother. He explained what happened. He'd been sick for several days when a friend finally intervened and demanded he go to the Naval Hospital. He detailed it in his concise, declaratory style.

"I had lost my appetite and could not sleep. My whole system was in a nervous or morbid condition. My mind was unbalanced. Reason had lost her sway. I became delirious and if this state had continued one more day, I would have been consigned to the spirit land."

Watts credited the Navy surgeons who tended him day and night. It felt like forever since he had "seen our people in Portsmouth," he told his brother, but the surgeons instructed him against going into town. In fact, the doctors knew Watts well enough to realize he'd see problems that needed attention and try to fix them. The only way he could restore his health, the medical experts said, was to leave town.

"If I cannot go to Portsmouth, I can be of little service and I might as well leave," Watts wrote. "I shall consider the matter, but it will be a struggle for me to desert them."

Portsmouth was so broken it was beyond the help of one man. Big plans were afoot to save the residents who remained. The mayors of Baltimore and Charleston joined with VERDAD and Philadelphia's Thomas Webster and advised relocating the town.

The idea was to move everyone to Fort Monroe at Old Point Comfort. For that, the federal government would have to sign off. If the government approved, it would still be questionable. How many were even well enough to get from their homes to the steamer wharves? What about the ones who couldn't?

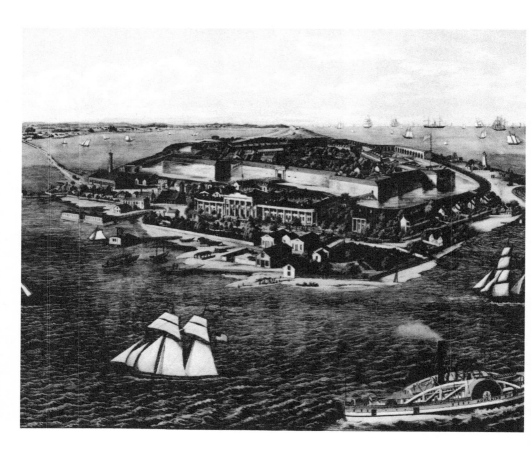

An 1861 view of Old Point Comfort and Fort Monroe from the Library of Congress.

CHAPTER THIRTEEN
The Dead and the Dying

O N Sunday, September 2, Reverend George Armstrong intended to hold a church service at First Presbyterian, if anyone showed up. That would be a few hours from now. He had again had trouble sleeping, thinking about the sick he had seen yesterday and worrying about his daughter Mary.

He rose early, wrote to a friend in Richmond, checked on Mary, had breakfast, and left the house to make his rounds of sick parishioners. Dressed formally for church, he nonetheless hustled down the street and headed toward a home on Main Street. He'd been to this house and many others so often that he had a mental medical chart for each one. A widow and two children from the house had died of yellow fever in the past week and a half. Three other children got the fever and survived and had moved into an uncle's house. When Armstrong visited yesterday, a woman and her deceased sister's three orphaned children struggled with the fever in the upper story of the home. A volunteer nurse from Charleston tended to them. Armstrong went inside, climbed the steps, and to his delight saw that the children were better. Their aunt was not.

"The aunt is breathing her last, and life is going out like a flickering candle in its socket," he thought. "All we can do here is to go and secure for her a coffin."

Seven or eight other Norfolk ministers would have been making similar rounds that morning, half a dozen or so in Portsmouth, so the scenes Armstrong stepped into were recurring on block after block, in house after house, every hour of the day. The ministers didn't risk their lives to remain in town merely to soothe the sick; they integrated themselves as part of the social safety net—finding a coffin, fetching a cup of ice, sending for a doctor, securing food, and making sure orphaned children were removed from a house and cared for. Doctors didn't have the time, and there weren't enough nurses.

Armstrong scooted from that house to another home four blocks away near the Presbyterian Church. He'd been here a couple of days ago, when he discovered every member of two families in the house was down with the fever. He'd stood at the door and beckoned a passing doctor to help.

"I have already so many cases in hand that I cannot conscientiously undertake another," the doctor had told him.

After leaving that day, Armstrong came upon a volunteer doctor from Savannah who had just arrived in town and recruited him to call upon the house. The doctor embedded himself, becoming physician and nurse to both families. Armstrong wasn't sure what he'd find when he went inside on this day. He was delighted to see that the two mothers had recovered, at least enough to care for their own children a bit, and the others seemed to be doing well. The main need for this house, Armstrong figured, was chicken soup from the Howard Association kitchen on Market Street. The doctor couldn't leave to get it, the mothers were too weakened, and the church elder who had been fetching soup in a pitcher was tied up at the bedside of his dying brother.

"I must get it for them today," Armstrong said, adding a soup run to his to-do list.

It was midmorning, and Armstrong had time for one more visit before walking over to the church. He'd been summoned just hours earlier to call upon this house, where the husband and wife had fallen ill with the fever. He was recovering; she was not. Armstrong thought hers was an unusual case; she had not had much of a fever, but she appeared to be delirious almost from the beginning.

Armstrong walked straight into the house. No one knocked anymore. In most houses, no one was well enough to come to the door. "Mrs. J," as Armstrong identified her, seemed fine to him physically, if her nonsensical conversation could be ignored. A volunteer doctor tended to her. The doctor, from New Orleans, had treated scores of yellow fever patients. Despite what Armstrong was observing with Mrs. J, the doctor told him she would likely be dead before morning. She had entered the toxic phase of yellow fever, known for bleeding gums, bloody urine, delirium, seizures, and eventually a coma.[154]

When Armstrong approached her bedside, Mrs. J smiled as though she recognized him and held out her hand. He took it, and her hand tremored so much that the minister couldn't keep his own hand from shaking. Her voice sounded "unearthly," sweet and lilting yet strangely hollow. Still, he thought she sounded fine until she spoke more. Then Armstrong noticed that Mrs. J was speaking about herself as if she were removed from her own body.

"She expected from the time the fever appeared in Norfolk that she would die of it," Mrs. J told Armstrong, referring to herself. "She had wished to live a few years longer for her husband's sake, but God's will be done," she said.

Usually not rattled by anything, Armstrong was unhinged by his visit to Mrs. J. He had not seen a case like this. Paying a visit was all he could do. Now, he had to get over to the church. It was time for morning service. He'd already heard that only his church and one of the Episcopal churches in town were having a service today—two out of ten houses of worship.

He stepped into the pulpit, gazed out over the pews, and counted heads. It didn't take long. Only twenty-seven people turned up at one of the three largest Presbyterian churches in Virginia. He knew everyone was there who could be, and the rest had either fled town or were sick, or with the sick, or dead. Still, Armstrong felt good to be there.

He asked everyone to move to the pews up front, then the usually formal Reverend Armstrong left the pulpit and stood among the congregation of stragglers. He led them in prayer:

"Remember our sick and afflicted parishioners," he asked, "that though absent from us in body, in spirit they are with us and their prayer and ours is one—that God would say to this wasting pestilence, 'It is enough.'"

By the second of September, scores were dying every day. The number was an educated guess. A passenger who arrived in Richmond on the steamer *Curtis Peck* said fewer than half of the doctors, maybe only one-quarter, reported their list of dead each day. The passenger said the Howard Association's statement that only twelve died on September 1 was laughable.

"There are about fifteen lying dead now, and no coffins to bury them," the passenger said. "Forty-two were buried Friday, fifty-five on Saturday, and sixty on Sunday."

The numbers matched VERDAD's reporting; the correspondent counted forty burials on Friday, August 31, plus nine who died after the interments. That was just Norfolk; another twenty-seven died that day in Portsmouth. Nearly thirty of the dead went unburied due to lack of coffins. Others were laid three together into makeshift wooden crates. Still there were more. For them, the Norfolk City Council appointed a committee to oversee the digging of trenches at Potter's Field, a place normally reserved for just one or two residents who could not afford their own burial.

Confusion over who was dead carried over into the newspaper reports. The *Dispatch* reported that the conductor of the Seaboard and Roanoke Railroad, a man named Daughtery, died. Days later, the paper ran an update, titled "NOT DEAD," and explained the mix-up. The conductor had written out a list of the deceased as a favor to the press. Daughtery signed his name at the bottom, where it seemed to indicate he was on the list.

"He is not only not dead, but is actively engaged in his office, which he discharges to the satisfaction of everyone," the *Dispatch* noted.

The toll hit doctors as hard as the general population: Two of the physician volunteers from Philadelphia died; four other doctors sickened and were taken to the Naval Hospital in Portsmouth. Winchester Watts was down sick, Portsmouth's Mayor D.D. Fiske still suffering, and Doctor William Collins of the Seaboard and Roanoke Railroad was incapacitated.

Collins was a mover and shaker who could have forsaken his hometown of Portsmouth to make his mark, but like Doctor John Trugien, he always came back. He studied medicine at the University of Pennsylvania, then returned home and built up a busy practice. A few years later, he was elected to the Virginia legislature, then became an auditor for the US Department of Treasury under President John Tyler. While in Washington, he began recruiting investors for a railroad: Collins aimed to rebuild an abandoned rail line to connect the Elizabeth River in Portsmouth to the Roanoke River. The line would expedite trade from western Virginia and North Carolina, opening untapped markets of tobacco and timber. As Norfolk writer William S. Forrest had called for in his dissection of the city's economy years earlier, the line would connect to other railroads to reach as far west as Memphis, Tennessee. It would pry open a cornucopia of trade. Collins reeled in investors, founded the Seaboard and Roanoke Railroad, and became its president.

Norfolk society had collapsed to the extent that acting Mayor N.C. Whitehead planned to establish martial law. New regulations would allow the city to seize horses and carriages for the physicians to visit the sick. The law also proposed to force Black people who were able, but unwilling, to serve as nurses.[155]

The 1855 Virginia epidemic would not shed more light on medical treatments or the mystery of how yellow fever spread, but it would be a defining moment for care. People noticed that victims seemed to stand a better chance of survival when tended to by a nurse, even compared to those treated by doctors.

New Orleans put a small dent in the nursing shortage when a man referred to as "the whole-souled and gallant Ricardo" arrived by steamer with ten nurses, whom he dubbed "the French artillery." Seeing the situation upon arrival, he promptly telegraphed back to New Orleans requesting twenty more nurse volunteers. Ricardo stationed the French artillery at the old City Hotel. He operated with military efficiency: When a request arrived for a nurse, he'd call out a name, and the volunteer would quickly stand up and dispatch to where needed.[156]

Even with Ricardo's troop of nurses and Whitehead's aggressive martial law, something more, something ambitious, had to be done. The *Dispatch* had pushed the idea of moving the remaining residents of both Norfolk and Portsmouth to a place safely away from the virus. The paper found wisdom in writings from a now-deceased English doctor who had been inspector general of military hospitals:

"To pen up the inhabitants upon the infected ground is to aggravate the disease 100 fold; and is, in fact, as cruel and absurd as it would be to barricade the doors against the escape of the people of a house that had taken fire."

On September 3, Hampton residents hosted a delegation from Norfolk and Portsmouth to work up a plan. Hampton sits across the vast confluence of the James River and Chesapeake Bay from the two cities. Its involvement was both benevolent and of self-interest. Clusters of Norfolk and Portsmouth refugees already filled the streets of Charlottesville, Richmond, Baltimore, and New York, where so many had fled that stores sold out of black muslin and crepe for mourning. But among all the places people fled to, Hampton absorbed the most. Refugees clustered there in makeshift villages in hastily hammered together wooden shacks set up wherever they found an open field.

The Hampton Committee began with an assessment of the current crisis, and its conclusion seemed both logical and stunning:

"Unless the population of the cities of Norfolk and Portsmouth be removed, one universal fatality must be the result."

"One universal fatality" was a proper way of saying that everyone left would die.

The committee resolved to appeal for help to the governor of Virginia and the president of the United States. It would send a delegation to meet with both men immediately. And it meant immediately.

Their other important act? To name a distinct committee to raise private funds to commission the construction of a lot of coffins. Word of mass burials, of graves dug as shallow as two feet, of bodies decaying in the hot Southern sun for as long as forty-eight hours before being put in a coffin, was already driving even more of the population to flee. Leaders came to recognize flight as a good thing, but they needed a safe common area where relief supplies like food could be provided.

After morning church service, Armstrong hit the streets again to resume making his rounds. He went into a house he'd been to the day before when he saw the two or three healthy members of the family worn to exhaustion from tending to five sick scattered in rooms throughout the house. Today, it surprised Armstrong to arrive and see that the critically sick were quarantined from the other family members. A volunteer nurse from Washington had arrived and segregated them, so the "death struggles" of the dying would not frighten the ones who stood a chance.

The nurse told Armstrong her first night had been horrible. The oldest, Ida, awoke in the middle of the night. She leapt out of bed, screaming, and bolted down the stairs toward the front door. The nurse raced after her and grabbed her just before she darted into the night. Ida told the nurse she'd had a nightmare that she was running from a monster that was about to catch her. Armstrong knew that the girl's frayed nervous system was the thing to fear. It was another critical duty of a nurse: to keep the patient quiet and calm.

"The shock to her nervous system is likely to prove fatal," he thought.

Apart from Ida, Armstrong thought the rest of the children would recover, and there was nothing else for him to do for that house today.

At the next house, he entered and stood face-to-face with a fierce-looking dog lying quietly in the foyer. Armstrong knew the dog and couldn't understand why it wasn't barking or coming at him. Then, he heard the wailing upstairs. The sound terrified the dog, Armstrong figured. The wife was sick, her sister the one screaming and moaning in pain, two children were sick but surviving, and the husband was alive. He'd burst a blood vessel in his face. When Armstrong touched his hand, it was cold like a dead person's.

"What can we do for this household? I know not, but to assist in having Mr. B removed to the hospital, and to secure a coffin for Eugene. Florence will probably not need hers before morning," he wrote.

The sun dropped below the horizon. Armstrong had been tending to the sick for more than twelve hours, and he had one more thing to do. He'd visited with a family the evening before, and a parishioner he called Miss Helen asked him to make sure she had a proper burial. At the time, Armstrong didn't see her having physical problems. He thought, and hoped, that her lifelong struggle with depression was at work. But she died overnight, joining three others from the family felled by the fever.

The entire funeral party consisted of two family friends who came to help with the children, a nephew, Armstrong, and the two men who brought the hearse. The two men brought her down the stairs in a coffin, and Armstrong offered a brief prayer. The hearse drivers had too much work to do to stand around for a lengthy send-off.

"Then, placing the coffin in the hearse, it is driven off to the cemetery at a rapid pace," Armstrong noted.

It was dark out when Armstrong finally walked home. Physically, he was worn thin. Mentally, he felt more defeated than he'd ever been. And he was perplexed, wondering why the God in whom he placed so much faith would let this happen—worse yet, make it happen. In a quiet moment back home, he again pleaded: "Wilt thou refrain thyself from these things, O Lord?"

The Hampton Committee didn't intend to leave the fate of the two cities in God's or anyone else's hands. The members left Hampton the day of their first meeting and headed straight to Richmond. In fact, it seemed they didn't send a telegraph asking for an audience with the governor; they just showed up. He was out of town.

They rambled around the halls of the Capitol and found George Munford, secretary of state of Virginia. Neither the governor nor Munford could give the committee approval to use Old Point Comfort to relocate the residents, but they did sit down with Munford and he offered one piece of help. Munford and the mayor of Richmond would ask the city's ministers to solicit contributions to buy a few horses and send them down on steamers. The doctors in Norfolk and Portsmouth could get to the sick more quickly if they had horses.

With that, the committee was off to Washington to meet with President Franklin Pierce. They got an audience with him that same evening, September 4. The committee chairman, Reverend John C. McCabe of Hampton, addressed the president. Not that McCabe had to exaggerate in the least, and he knew that Pierce would have been reading reports daily, but McCabe laid it on thick:

"Mr. President, physicians are falling at their posts; nurses are dying at bedsides; and the ministers of the cross of Christ as they stand at the couches of the sick and dying are struck down," McCabe said.

Unless God or, hint, hint, "the strong arm of men in power" do something to stop the dying, the two towns will be entirely depopulated, McCabe warned. The ports will shut. Ships will no longer dock at the Virginia wharves. The supply of barrels, shoes, ropes, cigars, guns, bricks, and hats will dry up.

Pierce listened, then spoke. He had anxiously read the daily reports from the Virginia port cities and sympathized. He'd been at a springs resort, spoken with the refugees there, and cut his visit short to return to Washington to see what could be done. He'd had several special cabinet meetings to consider options. He would sleep on the committee's proposal to remove the population to Old Point. He asked them to return at 8 a.m.

When the committee came back, Pierce kept them waiting for two hours. Then he had bad news. He could not turn over the military portion of Old Point Comfort, Fort Monroe, to the cities. It would be impractical or perhaps impossible to move fifteen hundred troops and their families to somewhere else as quickly as necessary.

Pierce reached out to McCabe. The president handed him a roll of bills. He and the cabinet had taken up a collection and gathered three hundred twenty-five dollars, today's equivalent of about eleven thousand dollars. They would collect more funds in coming weeks, if needed, Pierce said.

Disappointed, McCabe and the committee sought out Secretary of Navy James Dobbin and pleaded their case. Dobbin agreed to do one thing that was in his power: He would order the Gosport Navy Yard to put carpenters at work making coffins.

The committee, undaunted, wasn't done yet.

On the way back home, members stopped in Baltimore to meet with the mayor, a Know Nothing party leader elected the year before. Samuel Hinks and a few city councilmen put their heads together with the Hampton Committee members and developed a plan B. They'd erect a temporary town of refugees on Craney Island, a peninsula just downriver from Portsmouth that pokes out into the Elizabeth River. Hinks and the council vowed to supply four thousand tents and send volunteers down the Bay to pitch them.

And the committee decided to pitch their Fort Monroe idea to the president one more time. Moor N. Falls, president of the Old Bay Line of Steamers, thought Pierce's primary hang-up was how long it would take to remove the troops. Falls had a form of power in the mid-1800s that few men had. His Old Bay Line could move a lot of goods and a lot of people very efficiently. Falls flexed his sway.

Our steamers could move it all—fifteen hundred troops, their families, their equipment—in twelve hours, Falls told the group. The

Old Bay steamers could haul them to Fort McHenry in Baltimore or bases in Washington, Philadelphia, or New York. The president can choose the location.

The committee sent a follow-up telegraph to Pierce with the good news. He was not impressed with their resourcefulness:

"I HAVE ANSWERED the committee from Norfolk, and assigned reasons which I thought ought to be regarded as satisfactory. It pains me to be constrained to inform you that the proposition of your city authorities does not tend to remove the difficulties."

They would have to go with plan B, though many people, Armstrong among them, thought the effort was doomed from the start. Armstrong compared it to an Army ordered to retreat when the soldiers' platoon mates are lying wounded on the battlefield. "There are sick and dying in almost every family, in a condition which places their removal out of the question."

Despite the still-mushrooming sickness and death, the slightest sliver of hope emerged. The calendar had flipped. On September 5, a new weather front came in and tamped the day's high to seventy-four degrees. It wasn't autumn, but surely cooler days were coming.

Even with the sketchy medicine of the day, and the utter mystery of what propagated the virus, the nation's collective experience with yellow fever had found solid agreement on one thing: The epidemics stopped in their tracks after the first hard frost: white on the grass and the rooftops, frost on the pumpkins.

In Norfolk and Portsmouth in the 1800s, people usually awoke to fall's first killer frost sometime in the first two weeks of October. That would be a grueling month away, with each minute seeming like hours, and the epidemic had not even reached its deadly crescendo. But a cleansing cold was coming, for whoever could stay alive for the next thirty days.

CHAPTER FOURTEEN

ANARCHY

A YELLOW fever attack first sidelined Norfolk's chief of police, Captain Elias Guy, toward the end of August. Then, it sickened his whole family. The city got by without the chief for a while. There were still enough well people in town to notice when things went awry, and the vast body of supposedly do-gooder outsiders had not yet arrived. By the second week of September, though, law and order crumbled.

On September 1, the *Dispatch* hailed the opening of a new hospital in the thick of the original infected district, just two blocks from the riverfront. Formerly called City Hotel, it had been converted and renamed "Woodis Hospital," in honor of Mayor Hunter Woodis, who died two weeks before.

The *Dispatch* said the attentive care and skilled nursing promised the sick would stand a better chance of recovery. The Howard Association had even placed one of its best nursing recruits in charge of the hospital, a Mister Isaac Marks,[157] who had just arrived from New Orleans.

"A good corps of nurses are engaged, and Marks, 'a host in himself,' will be constantly in attendance and see that everything is done that can be for the comfort and convenience of the sick," VERDAD wrote.[158]

Within days, in addition to his organizational job, Marks began assigning himself a person or two to nurse. He took it upon himself to tend to a family of eleven in a house next to the hospital. The fever had already sickened and killed the mother and father. The father had entrusted a fourteen-year-old son with the key to a trunk holding all the family's jewelry and money. The boy took this grown-up responsibility to heart. When he came down with the fever, he tucked the key under his pillow.

Tending to the sick boy, Marks found the key. He assumed the boy was too sick to live, let alone well enough to realize Marks was robbing the family. Marks assumed incorrectly. The boy recovered, identified Marks, and spilled the details of everything that happened. Marks had stolen more than one thousand dollars in money and jewelry, worth more than thirty-four thousand dollars today.[159] He confessed and, in exchange for being allowed to go free, showed where he had hidden the goods.

Enter VERDAD:

"STRANGE TO SAY he was released. He is about five feet eight inches tall, dark complexion, curly hair, quick when spoken to; his address is very good. Pass the scoundrel around."

Along with doctors and nurses, con artists had found their way to Norfolk. Another charlatan nurse came to town and got placed in the house of a family with every member sick. He robbed them, then downed the brandy that the doctors had prescribed. Barely able to remain standing, the sham nurse accosted Armstrong during his rounds.

I have a letter of introduction to you from one of your Richmond friends, the drunken man told Armstrong. *Can you get me a place as a nurse with a family needing one?*

Armstrong stared at him. The man did not hand over a letter.

You had better leave our city as soon as you can find a way to get out, he told the drunk.[160]

With the city's police chief down with the fever, Norfolk appointed Franklin H. Clack, a twenty-seven-year-old New Orleans volunteer, temporary chief of police. His father was a former Navy officer with whom Norfolk leaders were familiar, and they were confident he could stem the tide of crime. His other task? To speed up getting people into coffins and to the cemetery for burial.

Clack had his hands full. As with all disasters, hucksters aiming to twist the chaos to their own advantage turned up in many different forms. Philadelphia Relief Committee Chairman Thomas Webster fended off the ones he could before they could leech off the cities' misery. In early September, a man named John Street contacted Webster looking for his blessing to pitch a remedy and "preventative of yellow fever" to Norfolk residents.

"I expect that any profit arising from the introduction of it to be mutual," Street told Webster, suggesting Webster could pocket a few dollars.

Webster flat-out rejected Street, even sending back his own letter:

"'PROFIT' in the distress of Norfolk and Portsmouth is not within the province of this committee's business."

At least Street was proper enough to ask permission to sell his snake oil. Most were not. An eighty-one-year-old doctor took out an advertisement for his own concoction, Hampton's Vegetable Tincture, "the great restorer and invigorator."

"Hampton's Vegetable Tincture . . . has shewn itself most powerful curative of NERVOUS DISEASES, in their various forms giving new life and vigor, restoring the shattered constitution and thus infusing hope in place of despondency," an advertisement in the *Dispatch* read.

Should yellow fever not be the issue, Hampton's Vegetable Tincture also boasted a fix for "Diseases of Urinary Organs, Coughs, Asthma, Bronchial Affections, Consumption, Scrofula, St. Vitus' Dance,

King's Evils, Worms, Rheumatism, Gout, Neuralgia, and multiple other ailments." Fret not, women: The tincture also worked on "the numerous and complicated derangements of the female system."

There was one criminal Norfolk authorities would no longer have to worry about. VERDAD was delighted to report on September 4: "Goslin, the murderer of Murphy, has died in jail with the fever."

The cities had collapsed into a new level of desperation, of hopelessness, of utter disorganization. If things operated, they operated in an entirely new and unrecognizable way. Every man, woman, and yes, every child had to fend for themselves. No exaggeration.

One day during his rounds, a street inspector named Zachariah Sykes came across children playing on a vacant lot. Three young, curly-haired kids romped around with each other, rolling on the ground. Sykes saw that they didn't seem to have bathed in a while, and their clothes were dirty and torn.

"Where is your father?" Sykes asked.

"Pa-pa is dead," one of the children told him.

"Then, where is your mother?"

"Ma-ma is dead too."

"Then who do you have to take care of you?" Sykes asked.

Mary, the Black woman next door, brings us bread every day, they told Sykes.

With that, he gathered the children up and led them over to the Howard Association, which would place them with the rest of the yellow fever orphans.[161]

In Norfolk, the Howard Association had invested relief money to convert part of Christ Church into an orphanage, including stationing numerous volunteer nurses there to organize and care for the children. So far, the fever had made orphans of two hundred seventy children. Richmond, Baltimore, and Philadelphia sent letters offering to foster the orphans.

Despite Philadelphia's leadership among all cities in supporting Norfolk and Portsmouth for the past three weeks, Webster didn't think it was enough. He saw in the two cities' daily acknowledgment letters a much greater need, even if they didn't specifically ask for much help. From what Webster could tell, Philadelphians could not fathom the depth of suffering in the two cities. On September 4, he and the secretary of the Philadelphia Relief Committee wrote and published a lengthy appeal. It amounted to a relaunch of the campaign.

Don't hold back contributing because it seems too late, Webster wrote. Don't think for a moment that the amount Philadelphia has contributed, not even added to what all other cities have pitched in, is enough. Norfolk and Portsmouth are not New Orleans, where the fever hits every year, where entire hospitals exist to treat fever victims, and where most doctors and nurses are immune. Norfolk and Portsmouth food is now bought in Baltimore and shipped down the Bay, he wrote.

Baltimore was even building and sending coffins down on steamers.

"Norfolk and Portsmouth are poor, unused to the fever. It has caused universal panic. Besides sickness and death, there is poverty . . . thus it will be seen that at least five times as much money in proportion to population should be sent to Norfolk and Portsmouth as would suffice for New Orleans."

In the week that followed Webster's letter, Philadelphians contributed $30,028, worth more than one million dollars today. It was a timely avalanche of funds, allowing the cities to order bread, flour, and other essentials and have them shipped in.

But frustration seeped into Webster's letters. His marvelous ability and determination to organize, document, and archive every contribution, to confirm that they'd been received, made him the right man for the job. And it drove him crazy when Philadelphia sent a contribution to the Virginia cities and he didn't hear back. On September 5, he wrote to Howard Association President William Ferguson pointing out that Philadelphia had heard nothing from Norfolk since August 27—no instructions about what supplies Norfolk might need, no acknowledgment of a donation.

"IF OUR EFFORTS to assist you are not up to your expectations, do not blame us," Webster wrote. "We want information, and you will confer a favor to this community if you will see that we have a daily report from Norfolk. We get it from Portsmouth.

Yours truly, Thomas Webster Jr., Chairman."

Crickets from Norfolk.

Six days later, Webster again wrote to Ferguson, putting the specific words he wanted to hear into the letter:

"IT WOULD TAKE but a moment to write 'Yours of____ with____ enclosed is received; send us more.'"

Still, no mail from Norfolk.

Webster didn't know the grim situation in Norfolk. Ferguson was down with the fever, as was James Saunders, Howard Association secretary. The virus had attacked N.C. Whitehead, Norfolk's acting mayor, too. Frustrated but still intent on the mission, Webster began sending duplicate letters to Ferguson and Simon S. Stubbs, a former Norfolk mayor.

Ferguson would be in and out of his sick bed for the next couple of weeks, keeping the Howard Association running as best as a yellow fever patient could. People would bring letters to him to read. Volunteers would find his house and report for duty. Webster found out about Ferguson's condition by happenstance, when one of his physician volunteers arrived by train in Norfolk on September 9. Doctor A.B. Campbell went straight to Ferguson with the letter of introduction that Webster provided. Ferguson read over the letter and said he had mixed feelings about Campbell being there.

"I'm both glad and sorry to see you," Ferguson told Campbell. "Glad because it shows that Philadelphia has kept up her interest in

Norfolk, and sorry because you will most certainly get the fever and we don't have the nurses to attend to you."[162]

"But I had the fever eight years ago," Campbell told Ferguson.

"Every physician from the North is now either sick or dead," Ferguson said.

Doctor Thomas Marsh from Philadelphia was lying ill at the moment, he said. Singleton Mercer, a nurse from Philadelphia, was sick in the hospital, along with three other doctors from Philadelphia, several nurses, and two doctors from Richmond. One Philadelphia physician, Martin Riser, was attacked by yellow fever, went home to Pennsylvania, recovered, and returned to Norfolk to help some more.

Since Campbell reported having had the fever years ago, Ferguson said he would not order him to leave without consulting with a group of eminent doctors in town. Campbell met with doctors from New Orleans, Augusta, Georgia, and Norfolk, who then consulted among themselves and reported back to Ferguson. The next morning, a man named Mite Olin, a volunteer from Augusta who had filled the void of secretary of the Howard Association, handed Campbell a letter to give to Webster. Just days after Howard Association Secretary Saunders went down with the virus in late August, his replacement, Wheeler, had sickened. Campbell could hand it to Webster when he returned to Philadelphia, Olin told him. The city declined his services.

"The sad experience of the past few weeks has proved to us most conclusively that every northerner who comes amongst us is doomed to fall victim, adding to the already heavy burden of grief under which we labor," Olin wrote to Webster.

Webster responded that Campbell had deep experience with yellow fever and other tropical diseases while working at the US Military Hospital in Veracruz on the Yucatán Peninsula. But he understood and would refocus on helping in ways the city requested.[163] Within days, the treasurer of Portsmouth's relief group, Holt Wilson, sent Webster a similar note:

"My dear and kind sir, send us no more of your people," wrote Wilson. They greatly appreciated the help, and they were grateful for the other contributions. "This is enough. Let this suffice—but spare your people."

Campbell didn't think his twenty-four-hour train trip was a waste. The four doctors he consulted with took him around and let him observe three hundred yellow fever cases and two examinations of the dead.

No one knew, or had the time to tally up, how many the virus slayed every day. Armstrong was one of the few still well enough to walk about the city and see for himself. Aside from visiting and caring for his parishioners, he was at the cemetery on most days, some days more than once. He and Father Matthew O'Keefe, the priest of Saint Patrick's Catholic Church, had agreed to take turns visiting the main cemetery, Elmwood, every night to pray en masse for that day's victims.

On September 5, Armstrong rode along with a newly deceased parishioner to Elmwood. It was nearly 5 p.m., the gravediggers had been shoveling all day, and yet dozens of coffins still awaited burial. He spotted the head gravedigger.

"How many graves have been ordered today in the city cemeteries?" Armstrong called over.

"Forty-three," the gravedigger said.

Armstrong walked over to Potter's Field. He saw two towers of rough boxes piled like firewood, as high as a man could reach to stack them. The boxes, hammered together from whatever planks could be found, were intended to hold just one person. These days, sometimes they held two, three, or four. One member of the Howard Association told Armstrong that a few nights ago, with not even makeshift crates available, the gravediggers had to wrap eight bodies in sheets and bury them together. The Potter's Field supervisor told Armstrong they would bury forty more there that day.

Armstrong also knew several Black people had been buried that

day; he'd helped their friends dig one of the graves that morning. He
guessed that ten Black people had been laid to rest, which bumped his
count to ninety-three. And that didn't factor in the Catholic cemetery,
where Woodis had been buried. Armstrong figured the daily death toll
was more than one hundred.

He stood and looked around the cemetery before leaving. He'd
been there many times when things were normal, before the epidemic.
Normal felt like so long ago now. In early September, the cemetery
should be quiet, and the lawn would stretch like a tight green sheet
tucked to the edges. He should have heard birds flitting and chirping
among the old cedars and elms. On this visit, he saw gravediggers near
and far throughout the grounds. Instead of birds singing, he heard
shovels scrunching into the dirt. Instead of a green carpet, it looked
like a plowed field.

"The city and the cemetery have changed characters," Armstrong
wrote. The city was quiet, somber, home to the dead and dying; the
cemetery full of activity and people hard at work.

During the first part of September, a mysterious skin-crawling
phenomenon emerged in the two cities. Swarms of insects appeared to
sail in from nowhere, drawn like magnets to the doors and windowsills
of houses. People described these flies, if that's what they were, as
smaller and narrower than most flies. Depending on the witness, their
wings were a glossy bluish-black or sometimes a muted yellow or
brownish orange.[164] Newspapers reported on their arrival. In previous
Southern epidemics, the plague flies had appeared as daily deaths hit
their peak. Maybe, residents thought, the outbreak was running out
of steam. The *Dispatch* ran an item on September 3:

The plague fly:

"IT IS A FLAT INSECT, with black body and red belly, and
has very large wings. In Portsmouth they were so thick in
the streets as to annoy persons walking and induced them
to place covering over their faces. The appearance of this

fly is generally considered a good omen, as it is supposed to devour malaria."

The *New York Times* described the plague flies as having red bellies when first appearing in the two cities and yellow bellies right before they disappeared:

"THE INSECTS are very much like mosquitoes, except with large wings, and their bites greatly inflame the flesh and raise great knots on it."[165]

Armstrong had been told that the appearance of the fly marked the deadliest days of an epidemic. The timing of the plague flies and an epidemic's peak were so synchronized, he said, that some people in often-affected ports like New Orleans "believe that this fly actually eats up the morbific matter which constitutes the most immediate cause of the disease."

Armstrong first saw them on August 31 and noticed them on September 3, 4, and 5. He recorded the dates in his notes. They had almost completely vanished by mid-September. Donning his scientific hat, he grabbed a vial, collected a few of the flies, and corked it up tight to look at later. He made detailed observations first: They looked like a blowfly, or shad fly, with the body being longer than that of a house fly.

Doctor friends from up north wrote Armstrong about the plague fly, asking for his observations and speculation about how and why they emerged. His thinking mirrored precisely how, several decades later, scientists learned that *Aedes aegypti* mosquitoes arrived in port cities and set them ablaze with the yellow fever virus.

"WE MAY SUPPOSE that this fly is a native in those countries in which yellow fever is an indigenous disease and ... multiply rapidly in those atmospheric conditions which accompany the rise and spread of yellow fever."

" . . . THAT THIS INSECT having been brought here in the hold of the *Ben Franklin*, perhaps in the egg or larval state, one generation lived in small numbers as to not attract attention, this imported generation has produced its eggs in vast numbers."

Armstrong was so close. Everyone was so close. The jigsaw puzzle lay on the table, only a few key pieces out of place, and they couldn't see the picture it revealed. It was just like Josiah Clark Nott had said: "Facts that are before us constantly cease to excite reflection."

At that moment in 1855, workers were nearly finished building the forty-seven-mile Panama Canal Railway, linking the Pacific and Atlantic oceans. Connecting the oceans had long been a goal, but the effort jammed into high gear to meet trade demands prompted by the California gold rush. Thousands of Chinese, Irish, other Europeans, and Americans surged into Panama for the horrendous job. They had to fill swampland, working at times in water up to their chests, and bushwhack through jungle to construct the railroad's bed. Cholera, malaria, and yellow fever sickened and killed so many workers that fresh laborers had to be continuously brought in. Even with that, at times, so few men were available to work that the railway company had to stop construction. An estimated twelve thousand people died.[166]

Across the globe at that same time, an allied army of the French, British, and Turkish invaded Sebastopol in Crimea in a move to evict Russian forces and secure access to the Mediterranean. A correspondent of the *London Times* wrote that the British Army in Crimea was more tormented by mosquitoes than "the shot of the Russians." The *Times* wrote that it is "mortifying to human pride" that man could tap the winds for power, blast tunnels through mountains, and dam rivers yet not find a way to control mosquitoes.

"They irritate us by droning their dismal songs in our ears, and then sting us to madness while they thrust their long bills into our veins and suck our blood," the correspondent wrote. The supposedly brilliant men who convened recently at the American Association for the Promotion of Science should have proposed ways to either exterminate mosquitoes permanently or for "neutralizing their poison. But science is dumb and helpless before the mosquito."[167]

The plague fly was yet another false flag that sent scientific discovery on a detour to nowhere.

That evening, after leaving the cemetery, Armstrong was tired but had a lot on his mind. His twelve-year-old daughter, Mary, had somewhat recovered from her bout of the fever, at least enough for Armstrong and his wife to send her to Richmond to stay with friends and revitalize away from the infected city. Mehetable, his wife, had struggled with the decision. Armstrong had seen enough death and thought it was the right move. He walked from the cemetery down to the waterfront. He continued out onto a drawbridge, where he could stand and look back at the city. It was a rare chance for him to pause and ponder.

Two dozen wharves cascaded down the riverfront, their warehouses labeled with owners' names in sharp white lettering: Newton's Wharf, Myer's Wharf, Woodside's Wharf, McIntosh's, Maxwell's. It was the same impressive commercial waterfront as ever, except Armstrong did not see a single person moving among the wharves. The ships that would be docked at the wharves year-round—and in early spring wait at the wharf heads five and six deep—were gone. The only thing he saw were the two masts of a fishing boat that had sunk at one of the docks.

"The only boat that enters our harbor now is the little steamer, the *Coffee*," Armstrong noted. "By her our mails are carried and all commerce done. Yesterday she came in with her whole deck piled with coffins." Mariners now shunned the Norfolk harbor as if it were "full of sunken rocks."[168]

Armstrong walked home a little more slowly than usual. He felt sad, more down than any time since the outbreak began. He understood that his isolation from normal human contact had seeped into his being. He was self-aware enough to know that he was depressed.

The sun had set, and he crawled into bed. As tired as he was, he couldn't sleep. He was anxious. His face tingled with sharp pain.

CHAPTER FIFTEEN
CLOSING IN

O
N Sunday, September 9, in Washington, DC, Reverend George D. Cummins climbed to the pulpit of Trinity Church to deliver a sermon honoring the sufferers in Virginia. Though readers of nearly any newspaper in the nation could find daily reports of the epidemic's devastation, they may have come away with the idea that this latest outbreak was on par with others they'd read about in the South over the past few years. Cummins stood ready to accentuate the uniquely horrendous devastation in Norfolk and Portsmouth.

The thirty-two-year-old Cummins was a traditional evangelical preacher who had no patience with the rituals and ceremonies that had invaded Protestantism. He'd later get booted from the Episcopal Church for his stance against what he saw as Catholic-style ritualism. He lashed back the way religious leaders had done for centuries: He founded a competing branch, the Reformed Episcopal Church.[169] The only ritual Cummins usually concerned himself with was pounding parishioners with bombastic words from the pulpit, and this day he was at the top of his game. He was especially hyped up, because the Norfolk church he headed for six years before becoming rector in Washington had now been converted to a home for the epidemic's orphans. For thirty minutes, Cummins rained the double threat of hellfire and eternal damnation upon the parishioners.[170]

Lesson one: The yellow fever epidemic came from God. Moses predicted in the Bible if people turned from God "the Lord shall smite thee with . . . a fever and with an extreme burning."

Cummins harkened back to the plague in Constantinople in the fifth century that wiped out tens of thousands; the bubonic plague that swept Europe in the 1500s; and the plague of London in 1665 that killed a quarter of that city's population in eighteen months.

"And now, nearer still does it advance, until we can almost catch the sound of the wail of the dying and desolation," Cummins intoned. "Without warning, the air of heaven became loaded with the seeds of death. The destroying angel was on the wing."

The Trinity Church collection plates that day gathered five hundred dollars, worth about seventeen thousand dollars today, to help the sufferers in Virginia.

Two hundred miles south in Norfolk and Portsmouth, people started seeing signs that the fever was abating. People still died by the scores every day, but the number of new infections seemed to be slowing. The *Dispatch* could not confirm it: An editor's note in the September 10 edition apologized for its "brief and unsatisfactory" account. The problem was, VERDAD had come down with the fever. Ever dedicated, he reported his own illness.[171]

"I WAS TAKEN down with the fever last night and am now confined to my bed. I passed a very bad night but feel better this morning and my physician thinks I'll be up in a day or two, my attack in his opinion being a mild one. I had selected a young man to continue my correspondence, but he, poor fellow, is down too.

Yours truly."

All the local newspapers had stopped printing, and with

VERDAD out of commission, reliable firsthand reporting was nearly nonexistent. It led to multiple false reports.

Annie Andrews, who had spent the past two months nursing victims, wrote a letter to the editor of the *Syracuse Standard* to say she had read accounts of her own death in newspapers. "If you hear it, I wish for my friends' sake you would contradict it as false," Andrews politely asked the editor.

She did offer fresh information: She wasn't sick, but she was worn thin. She'd been there for weeks on end, sat up late at night with patients most nights, and stayed up all night many times. Two of the best volunteer doctors had died just last night, she wrote:

> "THE CITY IS deserted and those who are here (except the Southern doctors and nurses) are sick," Andrews reported, then she shed new light on the optimism that the fever was waning. "They say the fever is on the decrease, but it is because it can find no more to kill."

She warned that if the refugees returned now, the influx of nonimmune people would surely spawn a new wave of the outbreak. She would have been correct. Most of the mosquitoes flitting about the two cities already harbored the virus.

Though the virus may have been waning, the death rate was not. Woodis Hospital had been open just twenty days and had admitted one hundred ninety-eight people. Even with experienced doctors, and nurses at the patients' sides, sixty-nine of them died: a mortality rate of 35.75 percent.[172] A *Baltimore American* correspondent did his own tally, counting two thousand dead in Norfolk—one of every three people who remained in town. "The great Plague of London only killed one in every ten of the population," he wrote.

The worst part was that as the waning virus thrashed and jerked like a fish trying to dislodge a hook, it seemed to be taking down more pillars of the relief effort, more of the folks who had kept the cities running.

Reverend Lewis Walke of Christ Church was down. Six ministers from the two cities were already dead. Doctor Robert Gordon, the health officer who had been deceived by the *Benjamin Franklin's* captain, had a dreadful attack. Reverend James Chisholm, who had helped move the Irish out of Gosport in late June, sickened and died. Two Methodist ministers, one from the White church and one from the Black church, died. Also dead or dying: the French teacher at the girls' school, the mathematics teacher at the boys' school, a former mayor, the helmsman of the steamer *Coffee*, the deputy postmaster, the postmaster Alexander Galt.

Winchester Watts, once he recovered for a few days, made his way up the Chesapeake Bay to Baltimore, then north to York, Pennsylvania. A surprising number of Portsmouth refugees wound up in York. It was an easy jaunt from the steamer wharf in Baltimore on the Baltimore and Susquehanna Railroad, which had been finished for nearly two decades.[173] Compared to the apocalyptic atmosphere in Portsmouth, Watts felt like he'd been lifted up and plopped down in the middle of a resort. He could hardly believe his easy life.

"A LOFTY CHAIN of hills encompass the town," Watts wrote to his brother, Samuel. "Splendid farms in the vicinity, and abundant crops. Some fifty or sixty people from Portsmouth have located here also many from Norfolk. I am staying at the best hotel in the place and pay $4.00 per week. The fare is excellent, good milk, butter, beef, lamb, mouton, poultry, vegetables, and fruit in abundance."

The Hampton Committee eventually carried out a plan, in a smaller way, to finally remove the population from the infected cities. Joseph Segar, a farmer in Hampton, offered his fields to establish an encampment not far from Old Point. Moor Falls, president of the

Baltimore Steam Packet Company, summoned two steamers and carted anyone who wanted to get away to the pop-up village. They set up enough tents to house fourteen hundred residents, with many large enough to hold a family. "All are watertight and comfortable. Let all come who can. Send them, we beseech you, that they may drink the pure and bracing air of this region," Reverend John McCabe, head of the Hampton Committee, wrote to the mayors of Portsmouth and Norfolk. People named the place "Camp Falls."

Only a few dozen took up the offer. They arrived with chickens, cats, dogs, and children who had the run of the vast field and their choice of tents. Most of the other residents in the ailing cities were too sick to move or had family members who were too sick.

Two Sisters of Charity tending the orphans in Portsmouth caught the fever and died. Thomas Webster's fear came to fruition when the fever attacked eighteen-year-old nurse Leonora Patterson, whom he had sent against his own instinct.

Doctor George Upshur, the man who had announced the first cases in Norfolk in July, caught the fever and slipped into the toxic black vomit phase. Upshur, known for his dry wit and courteous nature, sent notes with a courier to his fellow doctors and his Masonic lodge mates. He invited them to his funeral. "Would two o'clock be suitable?" he asked.

The orphans of the pestilence drew attention from everywhere. Schoolgirls in Philadelphia sewed one hundred eighteen pieces of clothing for the orphaned children and sent them down. A Jewish group in Charleston, South Carolina, began making clothing for them. Young girls in Richmond set up a flea market on Governor Street and raised fifty-seven dollars. A Portsmouth man bought enough books to supply an elementary school and donated them to the relief committee so the orphans could get a few hours of learning each day. Baltimore, Philadelphia, and Richmond each requested that the cities send the orphans to them. In fact, there was polite trash-talking in a competition to see who could love the children the most.

The *Richmond Dispatch* reported that to house the orphans, Baltimore had opened its doors to them in a a home normally occupied by foreign refugees. But Richmond should be the city to get the orphans, the *Dispatch* noted, because it had requested them first. "We trust they will be sent here. Besides, Richmond has a better place for them than the Baltimore House of Refuge."[174] Richmond found a large building about two miles from downtown that was being built for a Catholic college and began outfitting it for the orphans, who would undoubtedly be sent to the right place. The people of Richmond were aghast that children of Virginia would be cared for in another state. "Every power in Virginia should forbid it," the *Dispatch* correspondent wrote.

Richmonders recruited Reverend Thomas Hume, of the Baptist Church in Portsmouth, to be their liaison with the men running the Portsmouth Relief Association. Hume's assignment: Get Richmond some orphans. Norfolk had declined sending any of its children away. Howard Association President Ferguson said kindly but emphatically that while they might not have parents, they were at home, and they had support. After Hume made several trips from Portsmouth to Richmond and back, the city's pleading worked.

One September evening, the steamer *Curtis Peck* set out from Portsmouth up the James River to Richmond. Hume himself led a parade of twenty-eight bedraggled and homeless children down the gangway. They were from fifteen months to fifteen years old. For two of the children, no one knew their names or their parents' names. Two large carriages and several other hack drivers carried the children, Reverend Hume, Richmond committee members, and three Sisters of Charity across town to the repurposed Catholic college building. Women from Richmond had made five hundred dresses for them and stocked up on food, toys, and games. After a long, long day of travel, the Sisters put the children to bed right away.

By the second week of September, Norfolk and Portsmouth were still much like cities that had been set afire by an invading army. Lime powder believed to disinfect had been spread on streets, sidewalks, front yards, everywhere—and after every rainfall, it swirled in the puddles and runoff. To disinfect the air, some people wore small sacks of lime chloride necklaces when they went out in public. Trash piled up. Coffins sat on street corners stacked three or four high, ready for the next dead. One day, the fire squad responded to a street-corner blaze only to find out that someone had lit a large barrel of tar on fire to keep away the bad air.

Residents didn't really know what was going on anymore. Without its on-the-scene correspondent, the *Dispatch* got reports from a mishmash of unnamed writers. The posts were filed under the pen names JURY, OATS, GRAPHO, and FRIENDSHIP. One day, the *Dispatch* editor wrote a news item himself:

"The melancholy news of the death of Richard T. Halstead, the 'Verdad' of the *Richmond Dispatch*, will be received with sorrow and regret by the public who have been so deeply interested in his well-written letters."

Halstead left behind his twenty-nine-year-old wife, Frances, and three sons under the age of ten: William, Richard, and Warren.

Despite the continued grim news, a little bit of hope also crept in. Doctors and nurses who had immunity; the police chief from New Orleans; the few city leaders who had not succumbed to the virus; and the rare residents who were still well all began to find their footing. At least, they steadied themselves just enough to find a way to exist, to care for and house their own residents. People were downright gleeful to see someone who they knew had been attacked by the virus, who may have even been reported dead, out walking the streets.

It seemed, too, as Philadelphia's Thomas Webster argued, that people throughout the country had finally figured out that the 1855 epidemic wasn't the typical yellow fever flare that popped up in some port city every summer. Because of a triple threat—a population almost entirely of nonimmune people, an economy of laborers who only got paid if they worked, and a location where rivers fenced in the residents—Norfolk and Portsmouth needed more help and more money than any American city ever. And by mid-September, the financial floodgates opened.

Though Philadelphia and Baltimore shined, New Orleans kept pace with its generosity even amid its own epidemic that year. Yellow fever had yet again latched hold in New Orleans and would kill twenty-six hundred people. But that was almost business as usual for the Crescent City: With one hundred forty thousand residents, it had nearly ten times the population of Norfolk, and its population had been Darwinized to near immunity. New Orleans for the most part took care of its own that year. The city's by-now famous volunteer Ricardo, with his "French artillery" of nurses, had telegraphed from Norfolk for additional help. Two dozen more nurses heeded the call and arrived in Virginia to form another of Ricardo's regiments.

Two years earlier, when yellow fever paralyzed New Orleans, Norfolk residents had been among the first to send help. After all was said and done in 1853, New Orleans had funds left in its relief account. Now, the *New Orleans Delta* newspaper reported, the city wanted to empty the account and send all the money to Norfolk.

"They say the fund was subscribed by the whole Union to relieve their suffering in 1853," the *Delta* noted, "and the suffering now experienced in Norfolk and Portsmouth makes it their property."

The outpouring for the Virginia cities arrived from everyone and everywhere. The chief of Tuscarora Tribe Number 5, Improved Order of Red Men, in Washington, DC, took up a collection of twenty-five dollars to be equally divided between Norfolk and Portsmouth.[175]

Wilmington, Delaware, sent five hundred dollars.

E. Smith from Danville, Virginia, sent one dollar.

Doctor Joseph Schoolfield's brother in Huntsville, Texas, sent fifty dollars.

Weldon, North Carolina, heard the cities needed rice, so it sent a cask of it on the mail train.

An enslaved boy sent ten cents—all that he had.

A store owner in Massachusetts contributed fifteen thousand dollars. He was hoping to open a store in Manhattan soon. His name was R.H. Macy.

Funds arrived from Frederick, Maryland; Shepherdstown, West Virginia; Hillsborough, North Carolina; Columbia, South Carolina; York, Pennsylvania; Charlottesville, Virginia; Lancaster, Pennsylvania; and Boston. Boston had taken umbrage at all the attention Philadelphia received and raised three thousand dollars to add to the cause.

Webster, in Philadelphia, received word that the cities needed chicken soup for those recovering. He sent a nurse volunteer, who had been sent back to Philadelphia when more northern doctors and nurses were declined, to go out into the country and round up two hundred live chickens.

George Armstrong saw all the help as a powerful testimonial of the country's potential when everyone worked together. He took a shot at those agitating for the South to secede. Normally, his policy was to keep the pulpit for religious and spiritual thoughts and to keep politics out of it. "But I love my country, my whole country," he said. Armstrong wished those jumping up and down to cut the country in half would look at the unity demonstrated in the help for Norfolk and Portsmouth. A word of caution, Armstrong said, to the secessionists.

"Every kind word spoken, and every dollar sent us from the North, the South, the East, the West, is a witness for the existence of this slumbering power," he wrote to a friend in Richmond. "We are one people, and I have faith to believe God means to keep us one people."

After every few sentences Armstrong wrote to his friend, he'd stand from his desk and pace the floor for a little while. He was irritable, nervous. It was September 12, three days until his birthday. He sat back down and wrote more: He'd had a premonition lately, which he couldn't explain. It wasn't spiritual. He wondered whether he'd make it to his forty-second year.

For the past few days, numbness and tingling in Armstrong's face had kept him from sleeping. Once again, he crawled into bed and lay awake. Pain in his face radiated like a hot current. He got up and paced the room for hours.

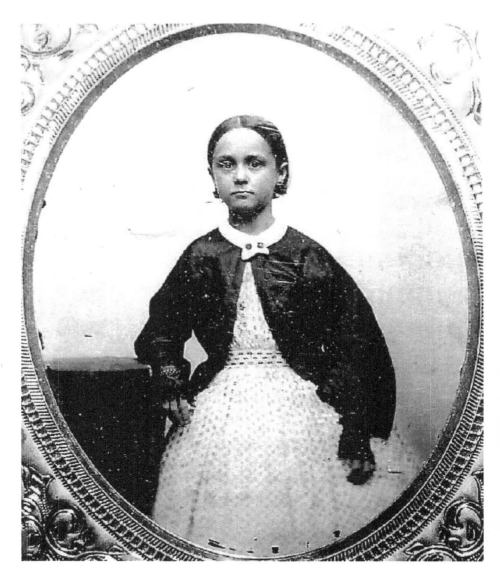

Grace Armstrong, courtesy of Walter B. Martin, Jr., via USGenWeb.

CHAPTER SIXTEEN
ARMSTRONG'S BATTLE

GEORGE Armstrong awoke the next morning with a dull ache in his head. September 13 had dawned as yet another hot summer day; the temperature only dipped to seventy-nine overnight, and warm, stuffy air filled the house.[176] Yet Armstrong had chills. Stubborn as ever, he wrote it all off to his lack of sleep. He ate breakfast, then left the house to visit the sick.

He followed a hearse to Elmwood Cemetery to say a prayer at the burial site, then realized he couldn't continue. He walked back home. He kept debating himself over whether he had yellow fever. He finally had to concede this was the beginning of it. He went back to bed. It was 11 a.m.

It was a terrifying yet not unexpected turn. As the outbreak moved from one part of the city and began to infect another, Armstrong had moved right along with it. All that time, he not only understood that he risked getting sick, but he also figured it was almost certain. The painstakingly bad timing was this: Armstrong had outlasted the worst days of the epidemic. He'd almost made it to a less dangerous time. Just as others had recovered, as the death toll began to slow, Armstrong vanished from the streets and hunkered down to fight for his life.

Though the fever was abating, it wasn't gone. The number of

daily deaths—twenty or thirty a day in Norfolk, ten to fifteen a day in Portsmouth—were now viewed with optimism. A month earlier, when infections and deaths increased daily, those same numbers had driven fear and panic throughout town. The events of the last two months had numbed everyone. On one September day, five doctors died: from New York; Montgomery, Alabama; Philadelphia (two); and Baltimore. A new correspondent for the *Dispatch*, who helped fill the gap caused by VERDAD's death, wrote that it was the largest mortality of doctors since September 5, when seven died.

Those who had suffered an attack of the fever and lived re-emerged from their homes to get supplies from the relief agency. "I see a great many walking the streets just up from the fever, looking as if the weight of a feather would knock them over," a correspondent who only signed his reports with the letter "F" wrote.

The *Dispatch* also received a letter from the editor of one of the Norfolk newspapers that had suspended publication, shedding light on what it was like on his last day of work. His staff members dead or sick, he could not find anyone to set the type. He stood at the printing wheel setting type himself and printing copies. After that, he had to put each copy in an envelope and handwrite the addresses, then get all of them onto the mail train. Nearly all his subscribers had left town and requested their papers at new addresses.

"I hope to never see such a calamity again," the editor wrote. "I feel five years older than I did two months ago."

A new *Dispatch* correspondent who signed his reports OATS dug deep for optimism in Norfolk. He found it one evening at 9 p.m. when he heard a familiar sound.

"The sun went down in cloudless glory, and now the moon shines forth clearly and mildly," he wrote. "It is a night of beauty—one of the great guns of that leviathan of the waters, the *Pennsylvania*, has just roared out loudly."

Armstrong's dedication to tending to the sick afforded him an advantage. He'd seen people lash against the fever's torment so violently that they made themselves sicker. He'd seen victims just give up. As with all things, even when besieged with the worst virus out there, Armstrong knew his life depended on a methodical plan. He knew he had to avoid flailing about; he had to ride the waves of torment. He had seen that the only food or drink needed was to suck on crushed ice. And he knew his mind might not be reliable. He moved a clock onto his fireplace mantel for an honest check on how long he'd been enduring the attack. He isolated himself from his family and stayed in his room to take on the virus alone.

He paced. He wrestled with his nerve-addled mind. He couldn't even describe how anxious he was, not from the thought of dying but from the virus's symptoms. At that moment, his body and the virus waged a battle that only one could survive. Viruses thrive at a person's normal body temperature. Armstrong's rising fever was his body's way of trying to cook the virus to death.[177] At that moment, the only thing he understood was that a "terrible nervous restlessness" taunted him to lash out in all the ways he knew he shouldn't.

"I'd rather die than lie still," he thought.[178]

Armstrong's mind drifted back to sometime earlier in the epidemic when he sat beside a sick young man at the peak of his fight with the fever. The man would aggressively throw his sheets off every few minutes. Armstrong would cover him back up only to have him flail around and fling the sheets off again. Armstrong did not understand why a person would work against himself like that.

"You must control yourself," Armstrong had told him.

"What do you think will be the consequence if I do not keep covered up?" the man asked, tension in his voice.

"Unless you can be kept covered," Armstrong said, "you will certainly die."

"Well, I must die then," the man said, tossing the sheets yet again.

Armstrong didn't understand the behavior then. He did now. Each day, each hour, his body felt more attacked, and his anxiety ratcheted up. He'd seen that medicines such as mercury chloride increased irritation of the person's stomach, which in Armstrong's opinion moved the victim a step closer to death. He stuck with treatments gentle on the stomach, a dose of castor oil followed by oil and warm water enemas. And he slowly chewed ice. He didn't know if this was the right medical path; no one did.

Mehetable did not inform her husband that as he fought the fever, their daughter Grace had come down with it, too. Mehetable tended to Grace. Mary was believed to be recovering in Richmond. With Armstrong and Grace perilously sick, Mehetable wished she had sent all their daughters to Richmond, where the air was healthful.

Amid the battle inside George Armstrong's consciousness—an angel on one shoulder, the virus on the other—his mind again replayed what he'd seen and heard that summer. Weeks earlier, he'd chatted with one of the volunteer doctors about a case. "I have never felt so powerless in the presence of a disease as in the presence of this one," the doctor said. "It scorns the skill of physicians."

Armstrong endured as the fever tossed and tortured him almost into a stupor for three days and nights. His skin was hot and dry, his body the most worn-out he could remember, his appetite gone. He lay in bed sweating, determined to keep covered, chills cascading over him. His heart thudded, his pulse seemed to skip beats and change rhythm. His eyes were bloodshot and teary. His head hurt, his neck ached. He applied a plaster of flour and cayenne pepper to the top of his spine to relieve the aching. His bed felt like it was made of bricks.

He pushed onward, somehow, to the evening before his birthday, his stomach burning. He remembered his minister friend Reverend Anthony Dibrell just before he died, saying that his smoldering, upset stomach was like the biblical term "the fire that is not quenched."

As he tried to lie quietly in bed, Armstrong's premonition returned—that he'd die before his birthday. The timing matched up. The fever had been coming on for nearly a week and had climbed to an intense peak. From what Armstrong knew, that was usually how long it took for the worst cases to come to a fatal, violently painful, end.

As the sun went down, he put an oil lamp on the mantel so he could see the clock. He moved to his bed and covered himself. He felt perspiration rolling down his body. Lie still, he told himself, or you'll die. He nodded off to sleep.

He awoke. Nervous. Irritated. How long had he been out? It must've been an hour at least. He glanced at the clock. Six minutes. It felt like six days. He stood and paced more. He put a small piece of ice in his mouth and walked a circle around the room. The restlessness never let up; it was the restlessness that was going to kill him. He knew he needed to be still, be calm.

But, oh, the irritability. He threw himself onto the bed and again fell asleep. He awoke and looked at the mantel. Ten minutes. Then he noticed the time. It was past midnight. He'd made it to his birthday. He covered himself up and went back to sleep.

While Armstrong fought the fever, the weather swung wildly. A cold front swooped down from the north, shoving aside the balmy Southern breeze that had been around the past few days. Low-lying clouds raced into Virginia, and for two days a nor'easter dumped rain and flung winds at the coast and battered ships at sea.[179] In Boston, three ships that departed port soon returned, the nor'easter having torn their sails off. Another ship got thrown onto the rock hazard, Toddy Rocks, on the way out to sea.[180] On Lake Michigan, the wind and rain of a surprise storm blinded the captain of the *Sebastopol*, an almost new two-hundred-forty-five-foot steamer that ran aground. It sat trapped as wave after wave dunked on the ship. Six people drowned.[181] "The storm was the heaviest ever known in that region," the *New York Times* reported.

Having shredded heavy canvas sails, with the might to lift entire ships, the northeast winds made quick work of Camp Falls. Armstrong fought for his life while pounding rains and gusts tore through the makeshift town. A few people who were too sick to leave were carted over to Joseph Segar's barn. Those healthy enough to move abandoned the campsite for good.

Richmond Dispatch readers soon learned that Doctor George Upshur had died of the black vomit. "Dr. George Upshur is no more," OATS reported. "The writer knew him well—intimately well, and was always a welcome guest at his fire-side. He was one of the warmest and at the same time one of the blandest gentlemen to be found."

The same day Upshur died, just four days after Armstrong made it to his forty-second birthday, Armstrong and Mehetable spent that Wednesday evening packing their belongings. Armstrong was better yet not out of the woods. The fever could still come back on him. "I am yet in a very feeble condition," he wrote, "by no means out of danger of a relapse."

With his battered body and his still addled mind, he knew he could no longer help his parishioners or friends. His family had not been willing to leave town, even for their own safety, if he stayed behind. So now he would go with them. At dusk, a courier knocked on the door and handed the Armstrongs a letter from Richmond: Mary had relapsed, and this time, her case seemed dire. Armstrong knew what that meant; he'd seen few over the past months who recovered from yellow fever once the virus returned in its toxic phase. Mehetable would not concede: She had nursed Mary back to health once, and her motherly touch could do it again. When they left in the morning, George would hunker down in Hampton with their daughters Cornelia and Grace and sister-in-law, Hatty; Mehetable would continue to Richmond to be at Mary's side.

Armstrong knew his family might "have the poison in their systems now," but he thought a cleaner atmosphere might result in milder cases. "At least for the present, I feel that the sooner we get away the better," he wrote.[182]

Just after midnight, he jolted awake. Wind whipped against the house. He hoped it wasn't another strong northeast storm because he thought the one over the past several days had accelerated fever cases again. He'd seen too many families finally decide to leave town, then get trapped when the fever sickened new members. He lay in bed worrying, unable to get back to sleep.

Around 3 a.m., he heard a door down the hallway creak open. Cornelia, the Armstrongs' middle daughter, had come down with the fever. A few hours later, the virus slammed Hatty. The Armstrongs weren't leaving town. They weren't leaving the house. They had waited too long.

On September 25, the doctors who had surged into Norfolk and Portsmouth over the past eight weeks held a meeting to determine which day they would return home. Incredibly, many of the nurses and doctors were now idle—at least for part of their time.

Doctor William Freeman, one of the first Philadelphia doctors sent south by Thomas Webster, proposed that the Howard Association get word to the residents who had fled not to return. Once it was safe, local physicians would make an announcement. The doctors also issued sanitation guidelines: Homes and businesses shuttered during the past two months should be opened back up by city authorities beginning October 10 to properly ventilate the sick air out of them before people returned. It would not be safe for the refugees to come back until "there is ice in the gutters."[183]

The doctors set October 1 as the day they could safely come back to their home cities. The committee secretary would write to the leaders of both cities to let them know. The toll on the doctors had been devastating: Even with many volunteer doctors from Southern cities—men who perhaps had immunity—twenty of eighty-seven of them got the fever and died. Physicians who died came from Richmond, Baltimore, Philadelphia, Washington, DC, New York, Georgia, Tennessee, Alabama, and Sussex, Virginia.

N.C. Whitehead, Norfolk's acting mayor, responded to the doctors on September 27. He expressed the city's deep gratitude and recapped how greatly their help had been needed. In just ninety days following Doctor John Trugien's treatment of the first cases in Gosport, the yellow fever virus had wrecked two cities beyond what anyone could have imagined before the summer of 1855.

"The annals of our civilization furnish no authentic record of a visitation of disease as awfully severe as we have just encountered," he wrote.

Whitehead explained that Norfolk's population, sixteen thousand before the fever broke out in July, had shriveled to an average of six thousand residents during the epidemic. Of those who remained, two thousand died—one out of three. Even among survivors, the fever had sickened nearly every resident who remained. Norfolk was now "a community of convalescents."

There was a period around the first of September, Whitehead noted, when "the evil seemed greater than we could bear." Corpses lay at street corners. The sick had no nurses. Some of the dead were buried with no family and no record of their death.

"Had we not received material aid from abroad, had not different portions of our country sent their heroic delegations of physicians, nurses and stalwart co-laborers, had not noble people volunteered to the rescue (to die, if need be, like Curtius for Rome) our people must have sunk beneath the burden of their agony," Whitehead wrote.[184]

While the two cities began to recover and make plans for residents to return safely, the Armstrong family was in the midst of an Old Testament nightmare. The fever suffocated Hatty's brain almost immediately, and she fell into a stupor. For the next two days, Mehetable nursed her sister and tended to Cornelia. All the while, anxiety gripped Mehetable because she couldn't go to Richmond to help her oldest, Mary. The Armstrongs' family physician, William Moore, knocked on the door; Armstrong had sent for him. The northeast winds continued, and that day the temperature would only rise to sixty-six degrees. Armstrong lit the fireplaces to warm the house. With two members of the house sick, six-year-old Grace went outside and played all day. Unsupervised, she wore herself out. She soon came down with the fever, too.

Hatty died quickly and mercifully. Cornelia and Grace were so weakened that Armstrong thought they might not make it. He was gripped with fear and felt powerless. "This must be the darkest day of my life," he thought.[185]

Then it darkened more.

Mehetable Armstrong might have mistaken the nervousness scrambling her thoughts as worry for Mary, or her sister's death, or Cornelia's and Grace's sickness. She felt worse and worse. When she broke into a sweat, she assumed it was from her busy nursing duties. Inside, her stomach felt hot. Armstrong knew the signs all too well: His wife now had the virus. Then Doctor Moore began showing symptoms of the fever and left for home.

Freeman, the doctor from Philadelphia, heard about the Armstrong family while at the doctors' meeting. He left and made a beeline for the Armstrong house. During Armstrong's daily rounds visiting the sick, he and Freeman had run across each other many times. Freeman had seen Armstrong's devotion, and he vowed to support the minister now. When he arrived, Freeman said if it suited Armstrong, he would bunk in the house and be their doctor round-the-clock. *"Give, and it shall be given to you,"* Armstrong thought.[186]

For a few hours, Armstrong believed his family might survive. Cornelia and Grace withstood the fever and began their path to recovery. The virus seized Mehetable much worse, but she wasn't so sick as to alarm her husband that her case might be fatal. But soon, when she began throwing up black vomit, Armstrong lost hope.

The next morning, he walked Cornelia and Grace down the hallway to their mother's room. She gave them each a memento and a dying wish: "In coming years, when you think of me, do not think of me as your Mother as in a grave, but as your Mother with Christ in heaven."

Armstrong ushered the girls out, then sat in the room with his wife. He tried to lift her spirits, and his.

"It will be pleasant to meet again with your mother," he told her.

"Yes," she said, "it will be pleasant to meet with loved ones again, but a more pleasant prospect than that is that I shall soon see Jesus."[187]

Armstrong had sat at the bedside of scores of people as they died over the past two months. He did it so often that, at times, he felt like he stood "upon some lands' end" that marked the border between the earthly world and the spiritual world. He saw hostile deaths, bitter deaths, sorrowful deaths, and tortured deaths. Now, he sat quietly with his dying wife. He absorbed the moment. He felt Mehetable moving from one world to another. She was at peace.[188]

Mehetable's mind stayed sharp until the last day. When her brain shut down and her thoughts stopped making sense, Armstrong saw it as a sign that she was being spared the searing physical pain that came to most victims of yellow fever.

Armstrong heard a knock at the door. He walked down the hallway to answer. A courier handed him a telegraph. Their daughter Mary had died. He didn't tell Mehetable. If she understood what he was saying, it would just bring her pain.[189]

The day after she spoke her last wishes to Cornelia and Grace, Mehetable Armstrong passed away around 11 a.m. Later that evening, George Armstrong and his two daughters rode behind the hearse carriage to Elmwood Cemetery, the burial ground where Armstrong had spent much of his summer.

As the sun set on that cool September day, Armstrong stood and prayed. He watched as the gravediggers lowered his wife into the ground.

BY EARLY OCTOBER, the sun lost its sizzle, and the weather cooled enough to spur residents to light their fireplaces early in the morning and at dusk. The cities were not yet in the clear. Mosquitoes reproduce best when the outside temperature is around eighty degrees, but *Aedes aegypti's* cycle keeps rolling, though more slowly, when temperatures drop to sixty degrees or even a little below.[190]

In Portsmouth, half a dozen new cases popped up each day, and four or five people died. One day, the *Dispatch* reported there were no deaths, a feat that had not happened since before the epidemic. Across the river in Norfolk, the city averaged eight new cases and eight deaths per day. Several of the dead were people who had fled the cities in early August, read reports that the fever had waned, and returned home too early. The difficult task, for leaders of both cities, was to convince refugees to stay away a few more weeks.

"I could hear of no new cases of the fever today, but is there anyone now in town that has not had it?" *Dispatch* correspondent J.V. wrote on October 1. "To have the disease rage with violence, we need only have more unacclimated persons. We must keep our citizens away until we have a good 'black frost,' as that is the only purifier of an impure atmosphere."[191]

Residents who had stayed behind and survived an attack of the fever reappeared on sidewalks and at markets. Though medical knowledge of yellow fever was beyond iffy, the survival of the volunteer doctors who were known to be acclimated provided sound evidence that past victims were bulletproof.

The Norfolk farmers' market appeared to reassemble itself overnight. Carts and wagons were loaded with a cornucopia of the fall harvest: apples, peaches, melons, beans, fresh meat, and fish. A schooner loaded with coal docked at the wharves. Three of the daily papers cranked up their presses again, and the *Southern Argus* put out word that it would commence publication on October 15. Make no mistake, scores of stores remained closed, and the cities looked like they had been ransacked, but residents could glimpse a hazy sketch of the before times.

Philadelphia Relief Committee Chairman Thomas Webster understood that the two cities would have needs for years to come. His committee continued sending supplies and funds south well into October. Webster, being a diligent person, had several items that he wanted to officially wrap up. He wrote to both cities: Was it true that they had thirty thousand dollars remaining? What had the cities done with the bodies of the Philadelphia volunteers who died? Could they even identify their graves? How would he dispose of the remaining funds Philadelphians had contributed? How many people had died?

Portsmouth Relief Association Treasurer, Holt Wilson, reported back to Webster. He didn't know how much they had left since they were still tabulating the debt the city had rung up during the past two months.

"I'm quite sure the graves of the Philadelphians can be identified. They were all marked," Wilson told Webster.

He also told Webster they had ample funds available for the expenses coming in, so Philadelphia could stop sending money. If it suited, they could pay the bills and send the remainder back to Philadelphia or transfer it to their fund established to care for the orphans. They also could set up a bank account that they would use to provide relief to other cities in coming years, when yellow fever undoubtedly would infiltrate and wreak devastation in a different port. With a small federal government, disaster aid came only from other states and cities.

Webster responded, "I agree with you in your views of the surplus funds that you have in hand. So far as regards our contributions, we do not expect you to return anything."[192]

Webster had a lot of questions because much like Matthew Carey after the 1793 epidemic in Philadelphia, he planned to quickly issue a report. Unlike Carey, he'd keep any personal opinions to himself. His query about the number of dead was a tough one: There were the deaths recorded by doctors and deaths added to the Registry of Deaths by relatives, then there was a black hole of information caused by utter chaos.

Doctor Schoolfield, the one who had treated Martha Fox outside of town, had been cobbling together a report for the past two months. He told Webster he had rounded off the numbers, but his report was "nearly absolutely accurate." Schoolfield sent Webster a chart of Portsmouth's sicknesses and deaths, the numbers of which would stun the most calloused heart:

POPULATION DURING FEVER
Whites: 2,200
Blacks: 1,800
Total: 4,000
Cases Whites: 2,100
Cases Blacks: 1,700
Deaths Whites: 890
Deaths Blacks: 95
Whites Percent: 42 1/3 percent
Blacks Percent: 5 1/3 percent

"All agree in saying, that there were not 200 persons who escaped an attack of all that remained in town," he told Webster.

Norfolk had a tougher time coming up with a solid number. Solomon Cherry, who had become corresponding secretary of the Howard Association after its president and original secretary died, said he could not give Webster the requested information. The organization's new president had been working on a list of the dead for the past several days, Cherry said.

"He requests me to say that 2,100 is about as accurate as he can make it," Cherry wrote to Webster. "Owing to the great consternation, confusion etc. about the time the fever was at its worst, no correct account was kept. We have the register kept by the keeper of our cemeteries, and we find 600 burials whose names are unknown."[193]

In any way it was tabulated, the fatality rate of the epidemic exceeded any death toll that a disease had inflicted on a population since the country's founding. One out of every three people who stayed in town wound up dead. The *New York Herald* calculated that, should New York be visited by a plague as deadly, at the height of its siege it would kill twenty-five thousand people a week.

As for the Philadelphia volunteers, Cherry said the Howard Association had bought four lots in Elmwood Cemetery. In one, they would bury the doctors who had died there. In a second, they would inter the nurses. The third would hold the orphans who would die in the future, and the fourth would be for members of the Howard Association. They would be honored to be the final resting place of the heroic Philadelphia volunteers, Cherry said. They would later erect a monument in the center of the four plots.

Webster handled the suggestion with his normal aplomb:

"YOUR INTENTION regarding them is proper," he wrote back, "but the wishes of the wives, mothers, and sisters of the deceased . . . is to bring their remains to be re-interred here, and to erect a suitable marble monument to their memory."

After those life-altering few days in late September, George Armstrong remained in town for a few weeks. He helped bury his friend Reverend William Jackson, pastor of Saint Paul's Episcopal Church, on October 4—another minister's "green mound" in the cemetery, as Armstrong had predicted. After that, he, Cornelia, and Grace boarded a steamer to Richmond so they could recover somewhere, anywhere else, for a few weeks. On October 6, *Dispatch* readers learned of Armstrong's arrival:

"The Rev. Mr. Armstrong brings with him his two little daughters, all of the family that remain—his wife, a daughter, and some of his relatives having died of the fever. He was very ill himself and narrowly escaped death."

It again seemed like the entire Eastern Seaboard was on the move, with the action emanating from Norfolk and Portsmouth. The volunteer doctors, nurses, and pharmacists boarded steamers or trains to head home, while supply ships, those who had fled, bankers, grocers, and shipbuilders steamed back into Norfolk and Portsmouth. The Old Bay Line of steamers restarted regular service on its Chesapeake Bay routes between Baltimore and Norfolk. The cities relit their gas streetlights.

On October 8, the nightmare officially ended. A *Dispatch* correspondent logged one of the most routine yet critical weather happenings of Norfolk's and Portsmouth's history:

"We certainly had frost today," wrote the correspondent who went by F. "It is now to be seen on the house tops, and upon the still unwilted grass and flowers that will soon show its effects. As this will be death to vegetation, so I hope it will be to the fearful fever that has robbed our firesides, made our hearts desolate, and peopled the graveyards."

It had been one hundred days since Doctor John Trugien diagnosed the first yellow fever cases in Gosport. To those who had lived it, it seemed like a lifetime.

On November 1, the steamer *Curtis Peck* eased toward its wharf on the Norfolk waterfront, loaded with scores of prodigal residents returning home.[194] People who had stayed at home hustled down to the pier to greet them. The refugees aboard the steamer applauded the residents. The battered residents cheered back.

Armstrong and his two daughters returned to Norfolk on November 6 after being gone for a month. The following Sunday, he walked to church to deliver a sermon and stepped into the pulpit. It was the first time he had been "with my people" in two months. He stood without speaking for a moment and scanned those assembled.

He saw that about half the usual number of families had someone there, and only three families were not clad in black mourning crepe. His gaze stopped at another cluster of pews: The Howard Association had brought to church the children it would be fostering for years to come. Sixty orphans sat in the pews, ranging from two or three years old to fourteen. Some were found alone, or with a dead parent, in their homes.

Wherever Armstrong's eyes paused, he saw empty seats, a ghostly placeholder for someone who had died. He figured the church membership he had helped build over the past several years had been knocked back a decade or more.

Throughout his sermon, he could not throw off the sadness.[195] Nor could he, a man who regularly wrote more than one thousand words a day, find a way to describe what he and the city had just endured.

"There are incidents in the history of this pestilence—incidents of which I was an eyewitness—which no one who has tried the capacities, or rather I would say the incapacities, of human language will ever undertake to put on record."

There are scenes in nature, Armstrong thought, that are so beautiful or so wrenchingly painful that the most gifted artist would never be able to convey them on canvas. No writer would be able to capture it. Language comes from words created to describe everyday life.

What the residents had just endured was not everyday life, except during the summer of 1855.

EPILOGUE

I N the fall of 1855, Norfolk and Portsmouth residents who had fled the epidemic swarmed back home. Steamers headed south from New York, Baltimore, and Richmond carried full passenger loads, then ran nearly empty back north to fetch the next group of refugees. People surged in as if the gates had been thrown open at a concert.

Imagine that Norfolk's population had dropped to four thousand by the end of the epidemic: Six thousand had stayed behind, and two thousand or more of those had died. Over a period of weeks, ten thousand healthy refugees joined them. It was the same over in Portsmouth: By the end of the epidemic, only two thousand remained, and now as many as seven thousand vibrant residents reappeared.

Markets reopened, with fresh fish, meat, produce, tobacco, shoes, and fabrics. In the end, George Armstrong had been right: God had scattered the residents to save them.

For the refugees and survivors, life in the cities that winter and the following spring consisted of only two things: Honoring the dead and trying to prevent whatever had just happened from happening again. Ever. They had a lot of work to do. No place in the young country's history had ever had to pull itself back from the brink of extinction like the twin cities now had to.

Memorial services and tributes published in the papers dominated daily life, much like they did in New York after September 11, 2001. The histrionic writing of the day did not likely soothe the hurt of those who had lost loved ones.

"The insidious disease fastened its deadly fangs upon him and his pallid cheek, dull eye, and languid step showed as he walked the street that his life blood had received the fatal poison," the *Argus* memorialized one victim. "He suddenly sank down, helpless and delirious, and was soon a sallow corpse."

The newspapers ran heartbreaking poems written by parents who had lost children and wives who had lost husbands. Every minister in town conducted a sermon recounting the despair of the epidemic and remembering the dead.

At year's end, Reverend Tiberius G. Jones, who had fled Norfolk when the fever first broke out, delivered what one newspaper described as "an eloquent sermon" at Free Mason Street Baptist Church. In his absence, seventeen members of his church had died.[196] Fleeing Norfolk during the crisis did not affect his reputation for long, as he suggested in defending himself from VERDAD's attacks. Jones gave the commencement speech at the College of William and Mary the following year. After the Civil War, when he again fled Norfolk for the safer ground of Baltimore, he became the second president of Richmond College, now the University of Richmond.

On February 19, 1856, firemen from three companies gathered in downtown Norfolk at Market Square and began a Sunday procession toward the Cumberland Street Methodist Church. After a few blocks, Howard Association members and the orphan boys they were caring for joined the phalanx. The orphans took the lead, followed by the association and its newest member, John Jones.

Jones was the enslaved man who, while constantly puffing a cigar to purify the air around him, spent every day of the epidemic in a horse and carriage hauling the dead to the cemetery. Often, he had been the only one at the scene and, by himself, had to shoulder the coffin into the hearse, drive it to the cemetery, and unload the victim at graveside. Unbeknownst to nearly everyone, Jones had suffered a severe attack of yellow fever and survived.[197] City residents had honored their word and, in exchange for Jones's heroics, offered to buy his freedom. Virginia law permitted slaves to be set free but then required them to leave the state within six months. Jones wanted to stay in Norfolk. He turned down the offer and remained a slave.

The Philadelphia Relief Committee had provided for the orphans' care. The committee invested the money that remained after the epidemic in a bank note that would churn enough annually to pay for their needs. In all, Philadelphians had contributed $1.7 million in today's dollars to help Norfolk and Portsmouth—the largest sum of any city in the country.

A larger problem was children who lost only their fathers and women who had lost husbands, Norfolk's mayor explained to the Richmond Relief Committee. That winter, widows of the epidemic and their children got by with small payouts from the Howard Association and handouts from friends.

"We have not less than three hundred poor widows, and some of them have five, seven, nine, eleven children," Mayor Ezra Summers wrote.[198]

In the 1800s, women had few opportunities for employment, assuming they could leave their five, seven, nine, or eleven children at home alone while they worked. The problem would linger as the decades wore on. Ultimately, the epidemic left many women homeless, especially those who had been widowed or orphaned. One was Mollie Hogwood, a yellow fever orphan, who worked the streets downtown as a lady of the evening and was said to have more diamonds than any woman "of her class" in the city.[199]

By the late 1800s, Norfolk wallowed in sin and revelry, with more than two hundred forty bars, gambling parlors, and brothels. A publication named *New York Town Topics* called it "the wickedest city in the U.S."

But during the winter and spring of 1856, Norfolk and Portsmouth residents had set out on a fevered mission to clean up.

They'd settled on the cause of the epidemic. They were convinced that Philadelphia's famous doctor Benjamin Rush was right and the fever was of "local origin." Leaders of New Orleans had determined the same thing after their devastating epidemic two years earlier. It all made sense: After an 1800 yellow fever epidemic in Norfolk, two doctors had authored an account and placed the blame on the filthy, undrained streets in town. During the five decades that followed, Norfolk became obsessed with grading its streets to slope down to the river and paving them to help the water drain.

Everyone thought that did the trick, until 1855 that is. In January 1856, *Southern Argus* readers were told of the fallacy in that thinking. The *Argus* argued that the city was not as well drained as it was in 1800. Norfolk had been built on a peninsula, which was naturally and efficiently drained by tidal inlets. The creeks snaked through the lowest of the lowlands and, twice a day, incoming and outgoing tides drained the smelly, malarious water out of the city more effectively than any manmade fill or culverts.

The new City Hall that everyone was so proud of? The *Argus* said the city's filling of low-lying wetlands to create a building site was a health nightmare. "The filling up of the marsh constituted one of the most bungling improvements in a sanitary point of view that Young America in the wantonness of his youth and folly ever perpetrated."[200]

The *Argus* was right. Old maps of the city show "Back Creek" paralleling the Elizabeth River and slicing through the entire town two blocks off the waterfront. A detailed 1851 map shows Back Creek dammed up by streets on its east side and walled off by the sparkling new City Hall to the west.[201] To this day, when a nor'easter or a thunderstorm hits, runoff floods the streets where Back Creek was filled. I lived in Norfolk for fifteen years and saw this scores of times. Despite human efforts to channel it, water returns to where water always was.

As the *Argus* noted, well-drained streets are great, but most rainstorm water doesn't fall on the streets; it lands on sunken lots and other low-lying spots. Since the land doesn't drain, the water stays there for days or weeks stewing in the sun. Back then, people knew that fetid water emanated smells that turned the stomach. They didn't know, however, that the stagnant water was an ideal breeding ground for *Aedes aegypti* mosquitoes.

Cove and Broadwater streets, the "made land" where City Hall was built, were the worst in the city. "Cove and Broadwater streets ought not to be allowed to remain in their present condition a week longer," the *Argus* editor opined. "THE LIVES OF THE PEOPLE ARE AT STAKE. THE PROSPERITY OF THE CITY DEPENDS ON PROMPT ACTION."

Clean lots, frequently picked up residential garbage, well-drained streets, entrails removed from farmers' markets, and covered cisterns were all forms of cleanliness that were next to godliness.

The cities had been saved, for now, by the thousands of refugees who came back after the first frost the previous October. But if they allowed another major epidemic to take root in 1856, no one in the country would consider Norfolk and Portsmouth to be commercially viable. Ships would stop coming, shipbuilding and importing and exporting jobs would dry up, and residents would move somewhere with a healthier atmosphere.

An immediate concern about the city's health was that residents who had lost loved ones wanted to recover their bodies to honor them. That winter, people found the mass burial pits and dug up the ground to look for relatives. The *Argus* editor ran a column titled "Don't Touch the Graves," where he laid out his case:

"The earth, impregnated with malarious atoms from decomposed bodies has been thrown up to the surface," he wrote. "The seeds of the pestilence which have been deposited beneath the earth's surface should not be upturned before the approach of another winter."

That, of course, was wrong, but it would be fifty years until it could be proven so. During the last half of the 1800s, yellow fever continued to lay waste to port cities. It's easy to forget that Americans were still pioneers in that century, and the settlers' primary mission was both simple and difficult: to stay alive.

Yellow fever epidemics in the five decades that followed 1855 occurred almost annually: Charleston in 1856 (two hundred thirty-eight deaths); Charleston, Galveston, Mobile, New Orleans, Savannah in 1858 (nearly seven thousand deaths); Galveston and New Orleans in 1867 (1,150 and 3,107 deaths). And many others: Key West; New Bern, North Carolina; Memphis; Pensacola, Florida; Brunswick, Georgia; Greenville, Mississippi. And on and on. No port city was safe.

Not until the turn of the twentieth century did the US government finally prioritize an all-out hunt for the cause of yellow fever. It became a priority for the nation's defense. In 1898, the USS *Maine* detonated in the Havana harbor, killing two hundred sixty-eight sailors. The United States declared war against Spain, Cuba's colonial ruler.

Ignoring two hundred years of knowledge about yellow fever, the US invaded Cuba in late June, its rainy, disease-laden time of year. The US quickly overran Spanish troops already devastated by malaria, dengue, and yellow fever: Out of two hundred thirty thousand Spanish troops, only fifty-five thousand were healthy enough to put up a fight.

The US lost fewer than four hundred soldiers in vanquishing the Spanish, but more than two thousand were sickened with yellow fever. Having overtaken the island, the US stationed fifty thousand troops there to hold it. Theodore Roosevelt, colonel of the only unit that saw combat, posted a letter to the secretary of war back in Washington about his troops' fate:

"If we are kept here it will in all human possibility mean an appalling disaster," Roosevelt warned. "The surgeons here estimate that over half the Army, if kept here during the sickly season, will die."[202]

President William McKinley announced the appointment of the

Yellow Fever Commission, made up of doctors James Carroll, Aristides Agramonte, Jesse Lazear, and Walter Reed, an Army pathologist and bacteriologist appointed the group's leader.[203] The commission started with what science had collectively learned after two centuries. The sum was nothing but a trail of breadcrumbs that went back six decades earlier with Josiah Clark Nott's insistence that an airborne gas could not cause yellow fever—that, instead, it spread like flying insects move, from place to place. At the same time as Nott, French physician Louis-Daniel Beauperthuy homed in on the *Culex fasciata* mosquito, now called *Aedes aegypti*.[204] As part of his argument, Beauperthuy overlaid the territory of *Aedes aegypti* mosquitoes and regions where yellow fever had repeatedly broken out. Though the areas overlapped, it wasn't scientific proof.

Three decades later, Cuban physician Carlos Finlay built on Beauperthuy's theory. Finlay recruited twenty people, assigned fifteen to a control group, and had the other five bitten by a mosquito "loaded" with the yellow fever virus. Three or four of the bitten subjects showed signs of yellow fever, and none in the control group did. However, Finlay's experiment wasn't tightly controlled: The subjects could have contracted the virus just walking around Havana, a city with frequent outbreaks.

In the late 1870s, a Scottish doctor named Patrick Manson discovered that mosquitoes, as Nott and others had insisted, could transmit disease. Manson showed that they could carry elephantiasis, a tropical illness that damages the lymph system and leads to enlarged body parts. Two decades later, in 1898, Ronald Ross, a British Army officer, demonstrated that mosquitoes transmitted malaria.[205]

Suddenly, after two and a half centuries of haunting torture, most of the clues about yellow fever's origins pointed in a similar direction: the mosquito. But it was still unproven. Reed, Carroll, Agramonte, and Lazear talked it over and concluded that there was but one way to prove their hypothesis once and for all. It would be controversial, and it would carry great risk.

"Personally," Reed said, "I feel that only can experimentation on human beings serve to clear the field for further effective work."

Carroll put even more skin in the game: "The serious nature of the work decided upon and the risk entailed upon it were fully considered, and we all agreed as the best justification we could offer for experimentation upon others, to submit to the same risk of inoculation ourselves."

That summer of 1900, Lazear took charge of caring for the mosquitoes, giving each its own test tube and letting them feed on yellow fever victims at a hospital in Havana. On August 16, he put a mosquito that had bitten a yellow fever patient ten days earlier against his own skin and allowed it to bite him. Today, we know that the yellow fever virus needs anywhere from four to fourteen days to develop after a mosquito bites an infected person. Lazear did not get sick from the bite.

Two weeks later, it was Carroll's turn. Within two days of being bitten by a loaded mosquito, Carroll began feeling sick, his skin yellowed, and his body temperature raced to 103.6 degrees. He barely survived.[206]

At the same time, Lazear convinced an Army private to volunteer for the experiment. Lazear allowed the same mosquito that had infected Carroll to inject the virus into William Dean. Dean came down with the fever six days later. His case was convincing: He'd been in an Army hospital beforehand, where there were no known cases of yellow fever; he'd arrived there straight from the United States; he sickened in the right window of time after being bitten.

Then, a loaded mosquito bit Lazear. He presented the bite as an accident as he was loading mosquitoes for other experiments, though many thought he may have intentionally allowed himself to be bitten. Either way, thirteen days after the bite, he was dead.

When Reed, back in the United States, heard about how the experiments were conducted, he was apoplectic. Before Lazear died, he wrote to Carroll saying his case would prove nothing. Lazear could have contracted the disease at or near the Havana hospital, where yellow fever cases were plentiful. "That knocks his case out," Reed told Carroll, "I mean as a thoroughly scientific experiment."

Reed and the commission decided to once and for all eliminate conflicting possibilities. They found a remote location and built two small wooden buildings. In one experiment, they filled the house with clothes, sheets, and blankets that had been dirtied by yellow fever patients. Three volunteers stayed there for twenty days, and none contracted yellow fever, putting an end to the "bad air" theory of disease transmission.

In another experiment, volunteers stayed in the same building, divided with screening down the middle. On one side, they let loose infected mosquitoes to buzz around among the volunteers; on the other side, the screen kept mosquitoes out. Only one volunteer sickened, one of those on the mosquito side.

By January 1901, the evidence had stacked up and all pointed to the same thing: *Aedes aegypti*. Reed, who would be credited as almost the lone hero for the discovery, praised Carlos Finlay for leading his team to the doorstep.

"It was Finlay's theory, and he deserves a great deal of credit for having suggested it," Reed said. "I suppose old Dr. Finlay will be delighted beyond bounds."

It was a huge discovery, but not until 1937, nearly four decades later, did Max Theiler and others develop an effective vaccine. Theiler, a South African virologist, was awarded the Nobel Prize for its development. However, the discovery that the mosquito carried yellow fever at long last gave American cities a villain—and something to try to eradicate.

In 1905, with yellow fever again breaking out in New Orleans, Norfolk's mayor summoned his health commissioners and residents to a special meeting and called upon them to take all available steps to "prevent the plague of the tropics from getting a foothold" in the city.[207] As with most efforts, from 1900 to modern day, the tradeoff for killing mosquitoes was environmental degradation.

A man named only as Lieutenant Shaw told the gathered crowd that to exterminate mosquitoes, a large amount of crude oil was being shipped into Portsmouth and Norfolk. Shaw explained that wherever water stood still, mosquitoes would breed by the hundreds, and in a tidal swamp like Norfolk that translated to millions.

If standing water could be drained, it should. In places where it could not drain, in cisterns, manure piles, damp cellars, and mudholes, residents would have to "treat" the water with crude oil. How much oil?

Two tablespoons would be ample for every fifteen square feet of water surface, Shaw told those assembled. This would not only kill the mosquitoes there at the time but would prevent any more from breeding in that place.[208]

Cisterns in a part of Norfolk called Atlantic City were a particular problem. Nearly every house there had a cistern, some no longer in use. Shaw said they would have to be treated with crude oil, then screened off to prevent mosquitoes from breeding in the future. Even if the cisterns were still in use, they should be treated with oil. The drinking water would not be affected, the mayor said.

There would be no danger, he explained. The oil would constantly stay on the top, and in most instances the pumps would take up water from the bottom of the cisterns.

But dumping oil into standing water would not end yellow fever's bullying reign. That would come from a simple invention prompted by the Civil War.

During the war, a Connecticut company that made sieves saw business suffer severely since it could only sell its product in the northern states. An employee at the sieve maker had an idea to sell more wire cloth: Paint it to prevent rusting and sell it as window screens.[209]

This new screening was first used to cover windows on trains to keep sparks, cinders, and dust from flying into passenger compartments. By 1869, when people knew they didn't like biting insects but didn't know mosquitoes carried disease, the *Chicago Tribune* was advertising screens for home windows:

"THE ANNOYANCES of spring and summer, such as flies, mosquitoes, dust, etc., can be obviated by using wire window screens manufactured by Evans & Co., No. 201 Lake street. These can be obtained at fifteen to fifty cents a foot."

Slowly, through the decades, even the crafty *Aedes aegypti* mosquito could not get into most homes to hide under beds and behind curtains. The difference was so noticeable that in a 1930 survey, *Journal of Home Economics* readers ranked window screens among their homes' most important appliances. Only running water and sewage disposal ranked higher.[210] But that fix only took hold in the developed world.

Malaria deaths are again on the upswing, jumping from five hundred seventy-five thousand in 2019 to six hundred twenty thousand two years later across the globe, *New York Times* reporter Stephanie Nolen wrote in a fall 2023 story. Her five-part series, dubbed "The Mosquitoes Are Winning" by the *Times* podcast, attributed the surge to mosquitoes' rapid genetic adaptations: They've developed a resistance to the very insecticides used to battle them. And a new species has transformed itself into an urban dweller, resistant to pesticides, tolerant of drought, threatening an additional one hundred million people.[211]

Even the developed world isn't completely safe. Climate change has allowed mosquitoes to expand their range, and in 2023 the United States experienced twenty cases of locally transmitted malaria in Texas and Florida and even as far north as Maryland. Dengue fever, an intensely painful illness once called "breakbone disease," has popped up in places like France and Florida.[212]

The year after the 1855 epidemic and his stay as a refugee in York, Pennsylvania, Winchester Watts, and a few other men, brought to Portsmouth the kind of freshwater supply Watts had marveled at in Pennsylvania. He helped found the Portsmouth and Lake Drummond Water Works. He died the following year. His cause of death was not listed.

Annie Andrews became an absolute heroine after the epidemic. In 1857, *Harper's Weekly* featured her alongside Florence Nightingale in a story titled "Two Noble Women." A few months later, the *New York Herald* published what was to be the first chapter of a book Andrews was writing: "The Heroes of the Pestilence; or, Glimpses of Norfolk as It Is." Apparently, she never finished that book. She married, had a son, James A. Upshur, who she raised on her own after her husband died.

On January 12, 1859, another sad procession snaked its way through the streets of Norfolk. The bodies of the Philadelphia volunteers had been dug up from their graves to be returned home. A man named Nathan Thompson, who helped collect relief funds, had taken a steamer south to supervise the transfer of the deceased heroes. Thompson's son, Andrew, a doctor, had volunteered his services in 1855 and died of the fever.

The male orphans, members of the Masonic lodge, and the Woodis Riflemen fell in behind a hastily assembled marching band. "The procession, moving slowly towards the steamer, presented a truly solemn scene," the *Southern Argus* wrote, "forcibly reminding many of other scenes witnessed when and where their heroes fell."

It would have seemed impossible in 1855 for any Norfolk or Portsmouth resident to ever forget the epidemic. But two years after the procession of martyred Philadelphians, the first shots of the Civil War rang out. Virginia became ground zero for the fighting, and the shifting tectonics of politics, economy, and everyday life seemed to wipe clean all memories of yellow fever.

In 1863, President Abraham Lincoln appointed Union General Benjamin F. Butler as commander of North Carolina and Virginia. Lincoln, with Congress's help, had suspended habeas corpus, the constitutional right for an accused person to be brought before a judge. Freedom of the press and freedom of speech also were denied. The Union seized telegraph lines, censored the US mail, and arrested newspaper editors. At one point, the *Chicago Times* criticized Lincoln's administration, and the government shut down the paper. All told, during the Civil War, military authorities arrested more than fourteen thousand civilians.[213]

By the time of his Virginia takeover, Butler had been nicknamed "The Beast" for his brutal reign in New Orleans. Upper-crust New Orleans women seemed to be Butler's main obstacle to controlling the hearts of the citizenry: They would leave streetcars and churches as soon as Union soldiers entered, teach their children to sing Confederate songs, even spit on officers. Butler reported that one woman dumped a bowl of "not very clean" water, likely a chamber pot, from a balcony onto an officer's head. Butler issued what became known as the Woman Order, which legislated that any woman who showed contempt for a member of the US military would be considered "a woman of the town plying her avocation." [214]

Then Butler brought his tactics to Virginia. He focused much of his attention on Norfolk, a strategically crucial place because of the shipyards, the Chesapeake Bay, Fort Monroe, and its proximity to the Confederate capital in Richmond.

When Union forces took over Norfolk, Armstrong stayed dutifully and defiantly at his post in the pulpit. He had seen national unity in the relief that came to Norfolk from both North and South during the epidemic, but now he chose a side. When a relative of Armstrong said he "would like to spit upon" a Yankee, Armstrong praised him from the pulpit. Butler sent for him. He chastised Armstrong, then sentenced him to solitary confinement at Fort Hatteras. At some point, Butler lessened Armstrong's sentence. The minister was assigned manual labor on a street-repair gang. Butler installed a minister from Massachusetts in the pulpit at First Presbyterian.[215]

As a writer, I've "lived with" George Armstrong for nearly twenty years, and I'm still not sure what to think of his behavior during the Civil War. In addition to his comment about spitting, he spoke words from the pulpit that hurt my heart to even read. His actions go against the grain of everything he wrote during the epidemic: that a united country was a slumbering power, that God intended the country to be one, that relief funds were a testament to this unity. The best I can say in his defense is this: Armstrong lived in the South, his parishioners were Southerners, and in the politics of the day, their city was invaded and lorded over by a general whose tactics were brutal. It was a horrible time. A person can be a hero in one circumstance and not in another. People and their moral decisions are complicated.

After the war, Armstrong returned to his Norfolk home. Over the coming decade, he noticed the city creeping out from its downtown core. With an eye on the future, he helped establish a ring of churches in the emerging suburbs. He retired in 1891.

Neither Norfolk nor Portsmouth ever created a memorial for the victims of yellow fever, though Philadelphia erected one in Laurel Hill Cemetery for its martyred volunteers. People in the Virginia cities who want to see evidence of the 1855 epidemic will only find it on a small marker in Elmwood Cemetery, placed there in 2016. Donna Bluemink, a local resident who became a volunteer archivist about the epidemic, paid for the marker herself and got permission to install it.

Without Bluemink's work, many of the details of the epidemic might have vanished forever. Unbeknownst to nearly everyone in Norfolk and Portsmouth, Virginia, Donna quite literally uncovered details of the history of the yellow fever epidemic that had been buried. For months, she reviewed plot records of local cemeteries, walked to where a grave marker should have been, and jabbed a shovel handle with an eight-inch metal point into the ground. If the spike hit something solid, she dug down until she found a grave marker. Then she photographed it for posterity and put it on a website with its inscriptions. She found hundreds of gravestones that had been covered and lost through the decades. Donna Bluemink is a true heroine of the epidemic.

The Reverend George Armstrong lies in Elmwood Cemetery, a place he became so familiar with during what he called "the Summer of the Pestilence." Near his stone are markers for his nephew, Edmund James, his sister-in-law Hatty, and his wife, Mehetable. His daughter Cornelia was also laid to rest there, along with his second wife. Cornelia's marker stands as evidence that the epidemic tormented George Armstrong longer than nearly anyone else. On January 20, 1856, Cornelia died. No records speak to her cause of death; the assumption is that she never fully recovered from the yellow fever attack. Whatever the reason, when the epidemic ended, Armstrong was left a single parent to his last living child, his daughter Grace.

His tombstone quotes First Corinthians and does not mention his work during the epidemic.

A craggy elm tree reaches its branches like arms above their graves, and in the summertime, shades them from the worst of the sun. Unlike the summer of 1855, the cemetery is quiet and peaceful.

ACKNOWLEDGMENTS

I N the mid-2000s, parts of Norfolk, Virginia, flooded due to two hurricanes making landfall nearby and the frequent nor'easters that roll across the tidal region. As a *Virginian-Pilot* reporter, I pitched in on the news coverage, but my personal life is what put me onto this story. As a result of the flooding, my neighborhood, Colonial Place, developed a rat problem. One night, I attended a civic league meeting to hear a woman from the health department offer solutions about how to control our rat population. With a neighborhood full of artists, writers, and university faculty, an audience member inquired about taking a humane approach. The health department woman, wearing a floral dress and looking like a soft-hearted soul herself, stared the questioner dead in the eye and said, "You can have a heart now, but you're going to have to kill them sometime." She also talked of driving a truck that sprayed chemicals out of the back to kill mosquitoes. At the end of the night, I approached her and asked why she was so obsessed with rats and mosquitoes. "Well," she said, "I'm sure you've heard of the yellow fever epidemic." I had, but like most people in Norfolk, only superficially. I decided to dig into it.

That's when I first found George Armstrong's descriptive letters, published as a book, *The Summer of the Pestilence*. I read his story, jaw agape most of the time. Armstrong made several references I wanted to read more about, so I called the history room of the Norfolk Public Library. "Would you like to speak to the archivist for that?" they asked and put me on the phone with a woman named Donna Bluemink. She, too, had become fascinated with the 1855 yellow fever epidemic and had spent the previous year finding original source material and transcribing it word for word. Each time I asked Donna where I could find a document, she patiently waited for me to describe it, then in a soft, direct voice simply said, "That's on the website." She had located scores of original documents about the epidemic and painstakingly transcribed them, making it possible for people who wanted to learn more about the epidemic to read first-hand what was recorded at the time. I can't thank Donna enough for her work that made this book possible. She's been at the other end of countless emails and phone calls, always ready to point me to a source to answer my curiosity. Over the past twenty years, she's also become one of my most cherished friends. Along with Donna, I'd like to thank Robert B. Hitchings, president of the Norfolk County Historical Society and archivist/historian of the Wallace History Room at the Chesapeake Public Library. While heading the history room at Norfolk Public Library, Hitchings stewarded the collection of materials by Donna and the staff related to the yellow fever epidemic. They are a testament to the value of public archives and libraries, without which history would be lost.

When I first heard about the epidemic, I was an enterprise writer at the *Virginian-Pilot* and set about to produce what became a fourteen-part series for the paper . I'd like to thank the paper's top editor at that time, Kay Addis, for creating a job that let me pursue my curiosities and stretch my writing legs. I'd especially like to acknowledge Maria Carrillo, my editor for that original series, who gave this book its first edit and has challenged and inspired me as a writer for more than two decades. That series left me with many unanswered questions; my search for the answers over the subsequent fifteen or more years formed the basis of this book.

Thanks also to my *Pilot* teammates at the time, Earl Swift, Diane Tennant, Denise Watson, and Lane DeGregory for cheering me on. From the bottom of my heart, thank you to Tom Landon and Beth Macy for enduring an early draft of this book, but mostly, for being my *family* these past several years.

I greatly appreciate that someone I met via a news story years ago, Cindy Williams, reached out even before I had a draft completed and offered to read over it for typos. I am beyond thrilled with the eagle-eyed and thoughtful work that my editor at Koehler Books, Joe Coccaro, performed in being the final set of eyes on this story and to Suzanne Bradshaw for her elegant book design.

There are a few people I wish could read this book who I would like to acknowledge posthumously: my buddies Scott Harper, Tim McGlone, Al Zay, and Skip Wood, who would all be proud that I finally wrote this thing; and my cousin Dale Edler who always asked, "Are you still working on your book?" Finally, my mom, Christena Widdowson Wagner—I wish she could read this work, but I mostly wish could see her granddaughters now.

And yes, thanks again to Bonnie Wood for her optimism that I would get this done; and to my daughters, Ava, Sadie, and Lilla, three of the wisest people I know.

ENDNOTES

CHAPTER ONE

1 *New York Times*, July 3, 1855.
2 *Report of the Howard Association of Norfolk, Virginia*, Philadelphia Inquirer printing office, 103. The relief groups that received aid from across the country each published extensive reports after the epidemic documenting donations, recounting the events that led to the outbreak, and exploring its causes. These reports were a critical source of information used to tell this story.
3 *Report of the Howard Association*, letter from Jonathan Bowen to the Howard Association, July 28, 1856. The Howard Association wrote letters to those aboard the *Benjamin Franklin*; Bowen, the ship's chief engineer, wrote back with his account of the journey from Saint Thomas to Norfolk.
4 *Report of the Howard Association*, Virginia, 104.
5 Centers for Disease Control and Prevention, "Yellow Fever: Symptoms, Diagnosis, and Treatment."
6 Author's note: Portsmouth officially became a city in 1858. For purposes of simplicity, I refer to it as a city, not a town, in this book.
7 Dr. Jari Vainio, *Yellow Fever*, Division of Emerging and other Communicable Diseases, World Health Organization, 1998.
8 Vainio, *Yellow Fever*, 16.
9 Erik Heyl, *Early American Steamers*, Mariners' Museum Library, Buffalo, N.Y., 1953.
10 Francis James Dallett, "Paez in Philadelphia," *The Hispanic American Historical Review*, Feb. 1960, Duke University Press, 103.

11 *New York Times*, "From St. Thomas," Jan. 9, 1855.

12 *New York Times*, "The Steamer Ben. Franklin – Yellow Fever, etc.," June 9, 1855.

13 *New York Times*, "The Steamer Benjamin Franklin at Norfolk," Jan. 20, 1853.

14 National Climatic Data Center, *Meteorological Register*, Fort Monroe, Virginia, June 1855.

15 J.H. Powell, *Bring Out Your Dead, University of Pennsylvania Press*, 1949.

16 *Report of the Sanitary Commission of New Orleans*, 1854. This report is staggeringly indepth. It ran 531 pages of small type and is three inches thick when printed out.

17 *Report of the Howard Association,* 102.

18 Josiah Clark Nott, *Report of the Sanitary Commission of New Orleans*, letter from Nott to Commission, 95-104.

19 William S. Forrest, *The Great Pestilence in Virginia*, 104.

20 Forrest, *The Great Pestilence in Virginia*, 15.

21 Forrest, *Great Pestilence*, 15.

22 *Report of the Howard Association*, 102.

Chapter Two

23 James Keily, *Map of the city of Norfolk and town of Portsmouth*, Rolin and Keily, Philadelphia, 1851. This is a beautiful map that allowed me to zoom in on specific parts of both cities and helped build scenes of places as the epidemic moved throughout the cities.

24 W.S. Forrest, *The Norfolk Directory*, 1851-1852, 16.

25 Steven Johnson, *The Ghost Map: The Story of London's Most Terrifying Epidemic*, Riverhead Books, 2007.

26 George Holbert Tucker, "Forrest—Norfolk's First Historian," Norfolk Historical Society, Chapter 42.

27 W.S. Forrest, *The Norfolk Directory*, 1851-1852.

28 *Virginiaplaces.org*, "Blue Ridge Tunnel."

29 *The History Place*, "Irish Potato Famine," 2000.

30 *The History Place*, "Irish Potato Famine, The Blight Begins," 2000.

31 *Learn History*, "History of Quebec and Canada, Irish Immigration, 1840-1896."

32 *The History Place*, "Irish Potato Famine: Gone to America," 2000.

33 *The History Place*, "Irish Potato Famine," 2000.

34 *The History Place*, "Irish Potato Famine."

35 *The History Place*, "Irish Potato Famine."

36 John David Bladek, "Virginia is Middle Ground: The Know Nothing Party and the Virginia Gubernatorial Election of 1855," *The Virginia Magazine of History and Biography*, Winter, 1998, 35-70.

37 Bladek, "Virginia is Middle Ground," 35-70.

38 Bladek, "Virginia is Middle Ground," 54, 55.

39 Bladek, "Virginia is Middle Ground," 35-70.

CHAPTER THREE

40 *Report of the Portsmouth Relief Association*, H.K. Ellyson's Steam Power Presses, Richmond, Virginia, 1856, 87.

41 *Report of the Portsmouth Relief Association*, 120.

42 National Climatic Data Center, *Meteorological Register*, June 1855.

43 Douglas C. Heiner, "Medical Terms Used by Saints in Nauvoo and Winter Quarters, 1839-48," *Religious Educator*, Vol. 10, 2009.

44 *Report of the Portsmouth Relief Association*, 122.

45 *Report of the Portsmouth Relief Association*, 167-171.

46 James Keily, *Map of the city of Norfolk and the town of Portsmouth*, 1851.

47 *Report of the Portsmouth Relief Association*, 79.

48 Bruzelius, Lars, *Bruzelius.info: The Maritime History Virtual Archives*, "Neptune's Car."

49 *Report of the Portsmouth Relief Association*, 81.

50 *Report of the Portsmouth Relief Association*, 81.

51 *Report of the Portsmouth Relief Association*, 87-88.

52 Mark St. John Erickson, "This week in 1862 – an Old Point Comfort landmark razed," *Newport News Daily Press*, Dec. 3, 2018.

53 *Report of the Portsmouth Relief Association*, 89.

54 *Report of the Portsmouth Relief Association*, 89.

55 *Report of the Portsmouth Relief Association*, 122.

CHAPTER FOUR

56 Powell, J. "New contender for most lethal animal," *Nature*, 2016.

57 Powell, J. "New contender for most lethal animal," *Nature*, 2016.

58 Jeffrey R. Powell, Andrea Gloria-Soria, Panayiota Kotsakiozi, "Recent History of Aedes aegypti: Vector Genomics and Epidemiology Records," *BioScience*, Volume 68, Issue 11, November 2018, 854–860.

59 Centers for Disease Control and Prevention, "Life Cycle of Aedes aegypti and Ae. Albopictus Mosquitoes."

60 *Report of the Portsmouth Relief Association*, 125.

61 Newman, Kira S., "Shutt up: Bubonic Plague and Quarantine in Early Modern England," *Journal of Social History*, Spring 2012.

62 Newman, "Shutt up."

63 *Report of the Portsmouth Relief Association*, 124.

64 *Report of the Portsmouth Relief Association*, 124.

65 *Meteorological Register*, National Climatic Data Center.

66 David Holmes Conrad, *Memoir of Rev. James Chisholm, With Memoranda of the Pestilence*, Protestant Episcopal Society for the Promotion of Evangelical Knowledge, 1856, 92.

67 *Report of the Portsmouth Relief Association*, 129.

68 *Richmond Dispatch*, "Yellow Fever," Aug. 14, 1855.

69 *Richmond Dispatch*, Aug. 2, 1855.

70 James Chisholm, Aug. 3, 1855.

71 Winchester Watts, letter to brother, Samuel, Aug. 4, 1855.

CHAPTER FIVE

72 Annie M. Andrews, "The Heroes of the Pestilence," *New York Herald*, Sept. 20, 1857.

73 Andrews, "The Heroes of the Pestilence."

74 Brown, Alexander Crosby, "The Old Bay Line of the Chesapeake: A Sketch of a Hundred Years of Steamboat Operation," *The William and Mary College Quarterly Historical Magazine*, Volume 18, No. 4, Oct. 1938, 389-405.

75 Andrews, "The Heroes of the Pestilence."

76 Andrews, "The Heroes of the Pestilence."

77 *Richmond Dispatch*, Aug. 1, 1855.

78 Andrews, "The Heroes of the Pestilence."

79 Andrews, "The Heroes of the Pestilence."

80 Barry Waugh, *Presbyterians of the Past*, George D. Armstrong, 1813-1899.

81 George D. Armstrong, *Summer of the Pestilence*, "Letter I," J.B. Lippincott & Co., 1856. Published as a book the year after the epidemic, Armstrong used his journal entries, notes, and remembrances to compile a series of twelve letters to his friend, William Maxwell, secretary of the Virginia Historical Society. In this book, I have referenced based upon the letter number.

82 Armstrong, *Summer of the Pestilence*, "Letter I."

83 Christopher McFadden, *Interesting Engineering*, "John Loudon McAdam: The Father of the Modern Road," April 5, 2021.

84 Armstrong, *Summer of the Pestilence*, "Letter I."

85 Chalhoub, Sidney. "The Politics of Disease Control: Yellow Fever and Race in Nineteenth Century Rio de Janeiro," *Journal of Latin American Studies* 25, No. 3 (1993), 441–463.

CHAPTER SIX

86 Butterfield, Lyman H., "Benjamin Rush: United States statesman and physician," *Britannica*.

87 J.H. Powell, "*Bring Out Your Dead*," University of Pennsylvania Press, 1949, 10.

88 North, Robert L., "Benjamin Rush, MD: assassin or beloved healer?" National Center for Biotechnology Information, *National Library of Medicine* (Jan. 2000), 45-49.

89 Powell, *Bring Out Your Dead*, 12.

90 Tulchinsky, Theodore H. MD; Varavikova, Elena, MD; Cohen, Matan J., MD; "A History of Public Health, Miasma Theory," *The New Public Health* (Fourth Edition), 2023.

91 Jim Bradshaw, *64Parishes.org*, "Saint-Domingue Revolution."

92 Powell, *Bring Out Your Dead*, 19.

93 Powell, *Bring Out Your Dead*, 20-21.

94 Powell, 45.

95 Butterfield, Lyman Henry, ed. *Letters of Benjamin Rush: Volume II: 1793-1813. Vol. 5596*, Princeton University Press, 1951.

96 Butterfield, *Letters of Benjamin Rush*.

97 Powell, *Bring Out Your Dead*, 300-302.

98 Katherine Arner, "A Creole Complex: Yellow Fever, the Atlantic World and the Formation of Early Republican Medical Culture," Institute for the History of Medicine, Johns Hopkins University, 2011.

99 Arner, "A Creole Complex," 8.

100 Arner, "A Creole Complex," 20.

101 Arner, "A Creole Complex," 23-25.

102 *Report of the Portsmouth Relief Association*, 116.

CHAPTER SEVEN

103 Winchester Watts, letter to brother, Aug. 5, 1855.

104 Chisholm, July 31 letter.

105 Chisholm letter.

106 *New York Times*, July 9, 1855.

107 *New Orleans Bee*, "Fruits of the New Orleans Quarantine." July 11, 1855.

108 *New Orleans Bee*, July 11, 1855.

109 *New York Times*, "Quarantine at New Orleans," July 9, 1855.

110 Armstrong, "Letter II," Aug. 13, 1855.

CHAPTER EIGHT

111 Armstrong, "Letter II."

112 Armstrong, "Letter II."

113 *Richmond Dispatch*, Aug. 8, 1855.

114 Chisholm letter, Aug. 1, 1855.

115 *Meteorological Register*, Fort Monroe, National Climatic Data Center.

116 Centers for Disease Control, "Mosquito life cycle, Aedes aegypti."

117 *Harper's Weekly*, "Two Noble Women," June 6, 1857.

118 Armstrong, "Letter II."

119 Andrews, "The Heroes of the Pestilence."

120 Winchester Watts letter, Aug. 10, 1855.

121 Steven Johnson, *The Ghost Map: The Story of London's Most Terrifying Epidemic*, Riverhead Books, 2007.

CHAPTER NINE

122 *Richmond Dispatch*, August 16, 1855.

123 *Officialdata.org*, CPI Inflation Calculator.

124 *Report of the Philadelphia Relief Committee.*

125 *Report of the Philadelphia Relief Committee*, Aug. 22 letter.

126 *Report of the Howard Association*, 63.

127 *Richmond Dispatch*, August 21, 1855.

CHAPTER TEN

128 Reginald Horsman, "Josiah C. Nott," *Encyclopedia of Alabama*, March 5, 2008.

129 *Report of the Sanitary Commission of New Orleans*, 1853, 5-7.

130 Jo Ann Carrigan, "Yellow Fever in New Orleans, 1853: Abstractions and Realities," *The Journal of Southern History*, August 1959, 343.

131 Carrigan, "Yellow Fever in New Orleans, 1853: Abstractions and Realities," 343.

132 *Report of the Sanitary Commission of New Orleans*, 1853, 101.

133 Eli Chernin, "Josiah Clark Nott, Insects, and Yellow Fever," Department of Tropical Public Health, Harvard School of Public Health.

134 Daryn Glassbrook, "The History of Yellow Fever in Mobile," *Mobile Bay Magazine*, July 28, 2021.

135 Glassbrook, "The History of Yellow Fever in Mobile."

136 Evan Bush, "How do mosquitoes track you?" *Seattle Times*, July 18, 2019.

137 Noah H. Rose et al, "Climate and urbanization drive mosquito preference for humans," *Current Biology*, July 23, 2020.

138 Jeffrey R. Powell, "Recent History of Aedes aegypti: Vector Genomics and Epidemiology Records," *Bioscience*, Oct. 31, 2018.

139 Jason Daley, "Swatting May Teach Mosquitoes to Avoid Your Scent," *Smithsonianmag.com*, Feb. 5, 2018.

140 Kenji Kikuchi et al, "Burst mode pumping: A new mechanism of drinking in mosquitoes," *Scientific Reports*, 2018.

141 Jason Daley, "How Mosquitoes Sneak Away After Feasting on Your Blood," *Smithsonianmag.com*, Oct. 24, 2017.

142 World Health Organization, "Mosquito control: can it stop Zika at the source?"

Chapter Eleven

143 *Richmond Dispatch*, August 23, 1855.

144 William S. Forrest, *The Norfolk Directory for 1851-1852*, 101.

145 Forrest, *The Norfolk Directory*, 99.

146 "The Church Awakens: African Americans and the Struggle for Justice," *EpiscopalArchives.org*.

147 Absalom Jones and Richard Allen, *A Narrative of the Proceedings of the Black People During the Late Awful Calamity in Philadelphia, in the year 1793*, 1.

148 Jones and Allen, *A Narrative of the Proceedings of the Black People*, 5-6.

149 Jones and Allen, *A Narrative of the Proceedings of the Black People*, 15.

150 *Richmond Dispatch*, Aug. 22, 1855.

151 *Richmond Dispatch*, Aug. 22, 1855.

Chapter Twelve

152 *Richmond Dispatch*, Sept. 2.

153 *Report of the Philadelphia Relief Committee*, 93. In fact, quinine was then and is now a treatment for malaria but is not effective against the yellow fever virus.

Chapter Thirteen

154 Leslie V. Simon; Muhammad F. Hashmi; Klaus D. Torp, *Yellow Fever*, National Library of Medicine, StatPearls Publishing, 2023.

155 *Richmond Dispatch*, Sept. 5, 1855.

156 *Richmond Dispatch*, "Progress of the Fever in Norfolk and Portsmouth," Aug. 30, 1855.

Chapter Fourteen

157 *Armstrong*, "Letter VI," Sept. 6, 1855.

158 *Richmond Dispatch*, VERDAD, Sept. 4, 1855.

159 *Officialdata.org*, CPI calculator.

160 Armstrong, "Letter VI."

161 *Richmond Dispatch*, Sept. 2, 1855.

162 *Report of the Philadelphia Relief Committee*, Sept. 11 letter from Campbell to Thomas Webster, Jr."

163 *Report of the Philadelphia Relief Committee*, letter from A.B. Campbell to Thomas Webster, Jr., Sept. 11, 1855.

164 Armstrong, "Letter XI," Nov. 13, 1855.

165 "Yellow Fever; The Yellow Fever in Virginia; Disappearance of the Fly," *New York Times*, Sept. 13, 1855.

166 Fessenden Nott Otis and John Cresson Trautwine, *Isthmus of Panama. History of the Panama railroad; and of the Pacific mail steamship company*, New York, Harper & Brothers, 1867.

167 "The Plague of Mosquitoes," *New York Times*, Sept. 5, 1855

168 Armstrong, "Letter VI."

Chapter Fifteen

169 Allen Guelzo, *For the Union of Evangelical Christendom*, Penn State Press, 127.

170 Rev. George D. Cummins, "The Pestilence, God's Messenger and

Teacher," Sept. 9, 1855. The sermon transcript is 3,550 words in length, which would have taken about 30 minutes to deliver.

171   *Richmond Dispatch*, Sept. 10, 1855.

172   *Dispatch*, "Report of the Howard Hospital," Sept. 18, 1855.

173   Jo N. Hays, "Overlapping Hinterlands: York, Philadelphia, and Baltimore, 1800-1850," *The Pennsylvania Magazine of History and Biography* 116, no. 3 (1992), 295–321.

174   *Dispatch*, Sept. 12, 1855.

175   *Portsmouth Relief Committee*, p. 280.

Chapter Sixteen

176   National Climatic Data Center daily reports.

177   *MedlinePlus.gov*, National Library of Medicine, "Fever."

178   Armstrong, "Letter VIII," Sept. 19, 1855.

179   National Climatic Data Center, September 1855.

180   *New York Times*, "Weather at Boston – Marine Disaster," Sept. 19, 1855.

181   *Milwaukee Daily Sentinel*, "Wreck of the Sebastopol," Sept. 19, 1855

182   Armstrong, "Letter VIII."

183   *Richmond Dispatch*, Oct. 11, 1855.

184   *Richmond Dispatch*, letter from Acting Mayor of Norfolk N.C. Whitehead to the volunteer doctors, Sept. 27, 1855.

185   Armstrong, "Letter VIII."

186   Armstrong, "Letter IX."

187   Armstrong, "Letter IX."

188   Armstrong, "Letter IX."

189   Armstrong, "Letter IX." Armstrong's letters indicate that Mary died before Mehetable, but death records and gravestones show them passing away on the same day, Sept. 17, 1855. There is no record indicating that Armstrong told his wife that her daughter died.

190   Joanna M. Reinhold, Claudio R. Lazzari, and Chloé Lahondère, *National Library of Medicine*, "Effects of the Environmental Temperature on Aedes aegypti," 2018.

191   *Richmond Dispatch*, Oct. 3, 1855.

192   *Report of the Philadelphia Relief Committee*, page 116.

193 *Report of the Philadelphia Relief Committee*, letter from Solomon Cherry to Thomas Webster, Jr., Dec. 18, 1855.

194 *Dispatch*, Nov. 1, 1855.

195 *Armstrong*, "Letter XI."

Epilogue

196 Library of Virginia, newspaper article found in Delany family Bible, Richmond, Virginia.

197 Forrest, *The Great Pestilence in Virginia*, 273.

198 Ezra Summers, letter from Mayor's office, Feb. 22, 1856.

199 Thomas C. Parramore, *Norfolk, the First Four Centuries*, The University Press of Virginia, 1994, 256-262.

200 *Southern Argus*, Jan. 19, 1856.

201 James Keily, *Map of the city of Norfolk and the town of Portsmouth*, Rolin and Keily, Philadelphia, 1851.

202 Max Hauptman, *TaskandPurpose.com*, "That time 200,000 U.S. troops spent an entire war on sick call," Oct. 6, 2022.

203 Michael McCarthy, "A century of the US Army Yellow Fever Research," *The Lancet*, June 2, 2001.

204 Ronald D. Fricker, Steven E. Rigdon, "Yellow fever: Discovering the cause and designing effective experiments," *Significance*, June 2020.

205 Fricker, Rigdon, 23.

206 Fricker, Rigdon, 23.

207 "Health Board Calls for a Cleaner City," *Virginian-Pilot*, Aug. 1, 1905.

208 "Health Board Calls for a Cleaner City," *Virginian-Pilot*, Aug. 1, 1905.

209 *Glessner House*, "Brief History of the Window Screen," Aug. 28, 2016.

210 Kris Hawley, "Screens: A Window to Six Degrees of Separation," *MarylandScreens.com*, Dec. 10, 2018.

211 Stephanie Nolen, "Mosquitoes Are a Growing Public Health Threat," *New York Times*, Sept. 29, 2023.

212 Nolen, "Mosquitoes Are a Growing Public Health Threat," *New York Times*, Sept. 29, 2023.

213   Mark E. Neely, Jr., "The Lincoln Administration and Arbitrary
      Arrests," *Journal of the Abraham Lincoln Association*, 1983, 6-24.
214   Alecia P. Long, "General Butler and the Women," *New York Times*,
      June 18, 2012.
215   Parramore, *Norfolk: The First Four Centuries*, 218.

Made in the USA
Middletown, DE
30 August 2024

60022798R00156